Smashing Through Th

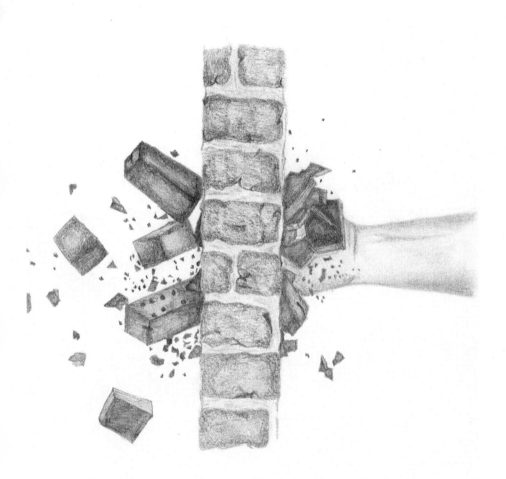

Cover Illustration by
Phoebe Adams

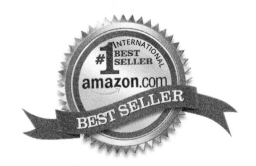
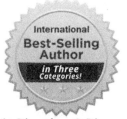

#2 in Disorders & Diseases
#10 in Death & Grief
#21 in Death & Bereavement

SMASHING
Through
The Brick Wall

Powerful true stories of cancer, rape, bullying & more leading to strength, rising up & conquering their lives.

Copyright © 2021 Rebecca Adams

ISBN: 9798740670614
Imprint: Independently published

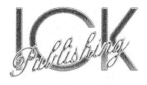

Published By ICK com. llc Publishing House©

Edited By Rebecca Adams & ICK Publishing
Cover Design and Book Design By ICK Publishing©

Cover Illustration by Phoebe Adams

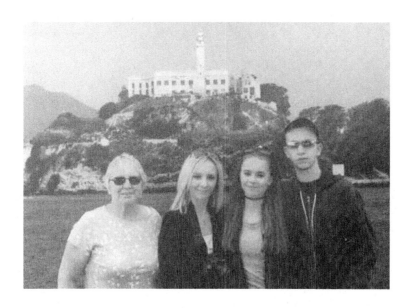

SMASHING
Through
The Brick Wall

Powerful true stories of cancer, rape, bullying & more leading to strength, rising up & conquering their lives.

Smashing Through The Brick Wall is a Compilation of 12 International-al Authors sharing their own real and raw personal life-altering stories.

This is a work of nonfiction. No names have been changed, no characters invented, no events fabricated.

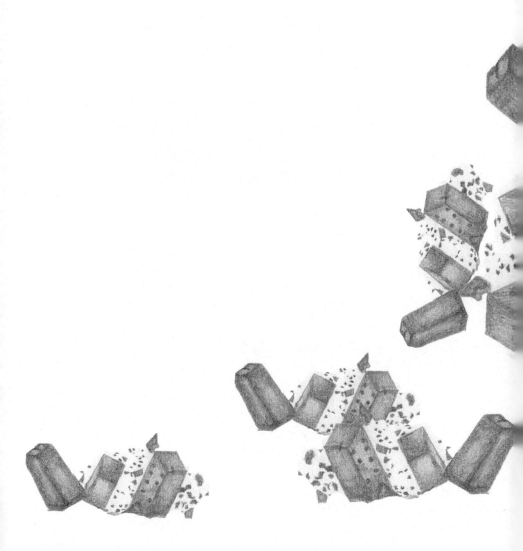

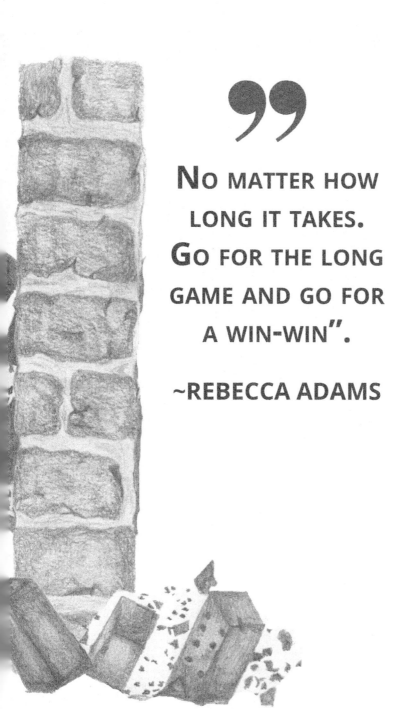

> **NO MATTER HOW LONG IT TAKES. GO FOR THE LONG GAME AND GO FOR A WIN-WIN".**
>
> **~REBECCA ADAMS**

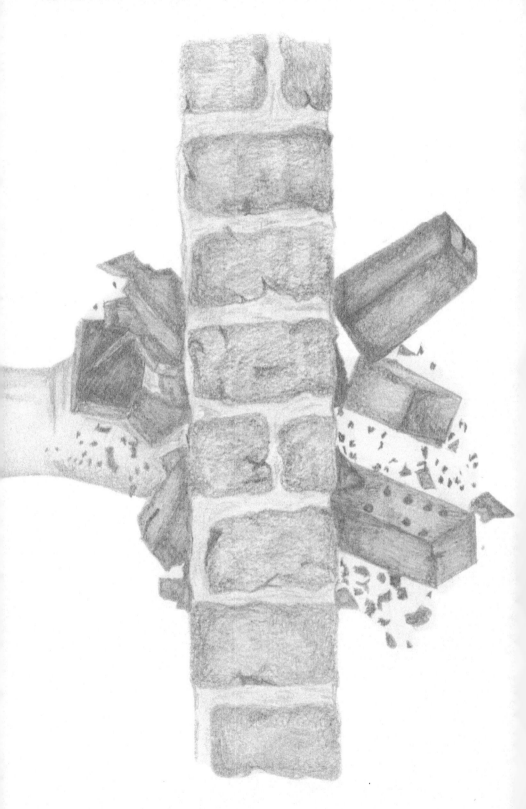

IN MEMORIAM

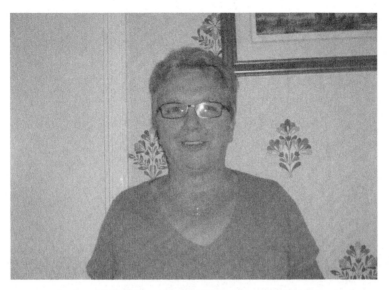

In Loving Memory of my beautiful Mum
Carole Arnold.
July 1949 - April 2021.

I am so blessed and proud of you Mum.
You always smiled throughout your cancer journey
and showed everyone how strong a person can be
regardless of the situation.

Thank you for being my Mum. I am so grateful to
have spent every single day with you along the last 10
months of your journey. Making memories, laughing,
smiling and enjoying our strong relationship as mother
and daughter.

Words can't describe how much I love you and what
you mean to me. You are a beautiful, inspirational,
courageous and brave warrior queen and I will always
love you dearly.

Be at peace and rest in love.
Always your daughter,
Rebecca. xx

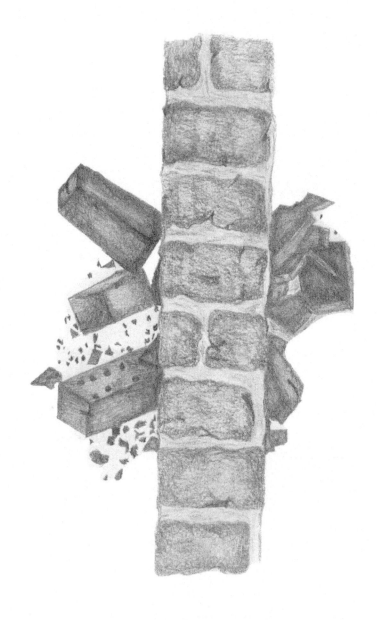

Foreword

As a Multi Award-Winning Inspirational Author and friend of Entrepreneur and International Bestselling Author Rebecca Adams, I am very honoured and privileged to be asked to write the foreword for this incredibly, inspiring book. Having written and published about a situation that happened in my own life some time ago, I knew this book would really touch my heart as it will yours.

Compiled by Rebecca and sharing her own story, Smashing Through the Brick Wall discloses real-life experiences by real life people speaking openly about the trials and tribulations of their personal lives, and in some cases the first time that they have ever spoken out about their challenges, nightmares, and fear of abuse, loss, bullying and much more.

I know just how difficult this would have been for each one of them to re-live their past. Bringing back memories that may have been buried for many years and not wanting to remember that time in their life, and for some, the pain and memories that still live with them to this day.

Sometimes in life we are faced with situations that have been through no fault of our own, even confine us like prisoners within our mind, which can be extremely difficult to know how to react. The authors in this book are stepping forward and sharing the most painful times of their lives with the intention that it will help and inspire individuals that may be going through similar things and to know that you are not alone.

Through adversity the authors have shown real strength and empowerment by releasing their feelings and emo-

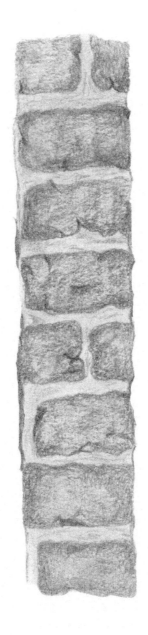

tions and allowing the reader to be part of their journey. It is not only courageous but inspiring, and I applaud every one of them that has taken part in this book, as they have shown real strength, bravery and truth, in sharing their story.

Smashing Through the Brick Wall is the second in a series of books where some of the most amazing, incredible people from all walks of life have come together in unity to support each other on their journey, encouraging others to speak their truth and setting themselves free from their own prison.

Whilst every situation in this book will be different, their story will be the same. Smashing through that brick wall is not always an easy thing to do but for these phenomenal women they did it and so can you!

Jenny Ford
Inspirational Author and Intuitive Writer
www.jennyfordauthor.com

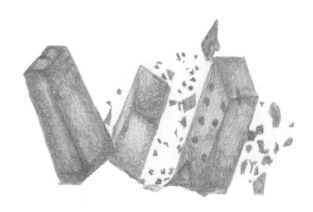

Content

Introduction...15

IN THAT SPLIT SECOND OUR LIVES CHANGED FOREVER 23
By REBECCA ADAMS

"The Big C"...39
By CAROLE ARNOLD

When a Family holiday takes an unexpected turn!........................51
By MARIA HARRIS

The EVER Changing You FALL, RISE & SHINE................................65
By IMANI SPEAKS

BUTTERFLIES & BULLIES..79
By NATALIE ALLANSON

The Secret Keeper... 93
By CHEVALA HARDY

The Pyramid Inside My Brain...107
By MICHELLE ROCHE

Making it out of the pit of despair...121
By CAROLINE BROWN

Up's & Down's of Parenthood..135
By MICHELLE NETHERTON

From Struggles To Success!...149
By LOUISA MOULTON

Content

Life can Change in an Instant......................................161
By LORRAINE FORD

SURVIVING THE UNEXPECTED..........................175
By LAKEISHA McGEE

Books Sponsors

Rebecca Adams...213

Maria Harris..215

Jenny Ford 217

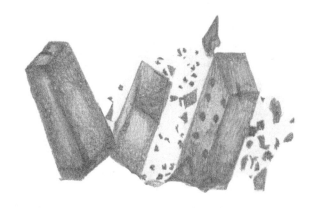

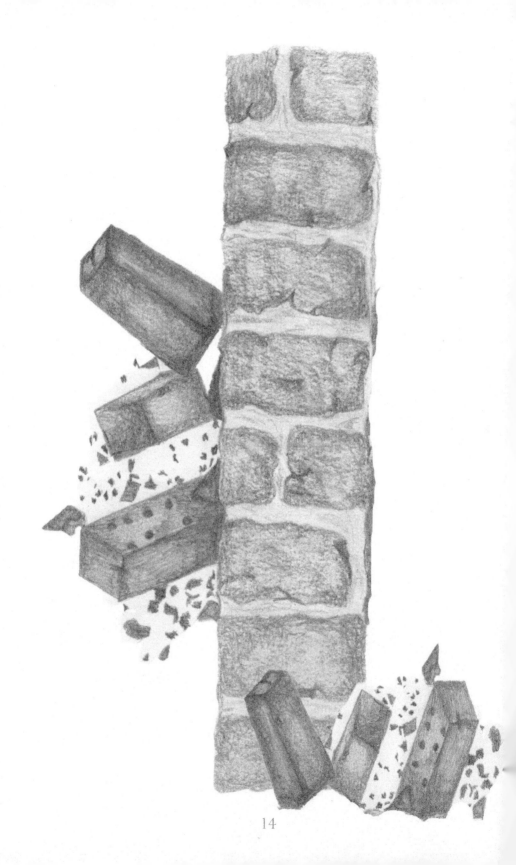

Introduction

I live a life full of high frequency gratitude for absolutely everyone and everything in my life. No matter how big or small things are – the ripple effect is huge and can impact many. I encourage you to do the same.

So, this is why I dedicate this book to you, the reader. Thank you so much, in advance, for reading this book because it's full of incredible real-life stories that may make you count your blessings even more than what you do already and help you see things differently too.

This book is for anyone who has been faced with their own brick wall – whether personally or professionally. The bricks may feel as though they are surrounding you, rising higher and you can't see a way through – know that there is always a way. Mindset is paramount in this completely as it's what you listen to and who you listen to which influences you more than you know.

The journey of your life is going to be full of ups and downs, trials and tribulations, and also on the flip side your life will be full of happiness, kindness, love, joy, laughter and amazing moments. The sad, dark and testing times will help you to rise up and be stronger but also help you to appreciate all of the wonderful and incredible things and people that can happen in your life too. The balance is there to help you to stay humble and grounded.

The bricks that may make up your brick wall could have lots of words on them like failure, fat, thick, stupid, ugly, pathetic (and lots of other toxic words!) BUT... you are in control.

You can knock each brick down one at a time!

To keep your spirit alive whenever you are facing brick walls is about taking each 5 minutes as it is, going into the faith of yourself or whatever you believe in and know that you can most definitely come through the other side.

I have a 4-step process for you:

1. Acknowledge
2. Deal
3. Heal
4. Move Forward

You have to Acknowledge whatever has gone on or is going on in your life and see it for what it is. Be honest with yourself and see it from all angles. Stay true to you.

Dealing with the situation is the most testing because you may have negative emotions towards it and seeing it from truth and properly dealing with it can take a while so get support from the right people who can give you amazing truthful advice (not just the people who will tell you what you want to hear). Take your time with this step. It may take a while.

Healing can take weeks, months or even years. Be gentle with yourself and do techniques that work for you in order to fully heal from the situation. Examples can include yoga, journaling, mindset work, listening to music, meditation, driving, the gym, prayer, travel and loads more. Do what will make your heart and soul align and sing to you.

The final step is Moving Forward with your life in whatever form that may be for you. No-one knows you but you can't leapfrog any of these steps so please don't try to. Take your time because the best work is done from the inside out.

A fully healed person's energy is radiant and powerful and will glow. Breaking free from whatever negative situation has happened or may have been holding you back is true freedom for you.

Embracing both your feminine and masculine energy is going to help too, so get to know what is more dominant for you and then learn to nurture the other energy. Masculine energy is all about taking action and getting things done whereas the Feminine energy is about resting, relaxing and taking time out. Finding a healthy balance is definitely the way to go – in all arenas of your life.

You may feel like you have had so many brick walls in your life to knock down that you're on an assault course. Know that each one is making you wiser and stronger than ever before and you can also inspire others who may be going through your situation.

You are not alone so please know that, and always reach out to people. Friends, family, professionals – whoever you need to and do not be ashamed, fearful or embarrassed either. Don't feel "less than" or have a "lack of" attitude or mindset because there are so many people who have been where you have been or know what you are going through and they will have amazing wisdom to share.

No-one ever knows what someone is going through behind closed doors. You can change someone's day or outlook on life with a smile or a word. YOU have the power to transform so many lives, starting with your own when you get out of your own way and release all of the icky, negative emotions, feelings, thoughts, issues and drama in your life. EFT (tapping) is a fabulous clearing technique that you can use.

The one thing I do is that I nip things in the bud straight away – no faffing about because it doesn't feel good in my gut and that's my inner compass warning me about stuff. It's always right too, in every scenario in my entire life so far!

Every day, keep showing up and keep your head held high to know that you can come through the other side for whatever your scenario is.

A quote I've said for years is:

"If you're given a brick wall - get round it, through it, under it or over it – get to the other side".

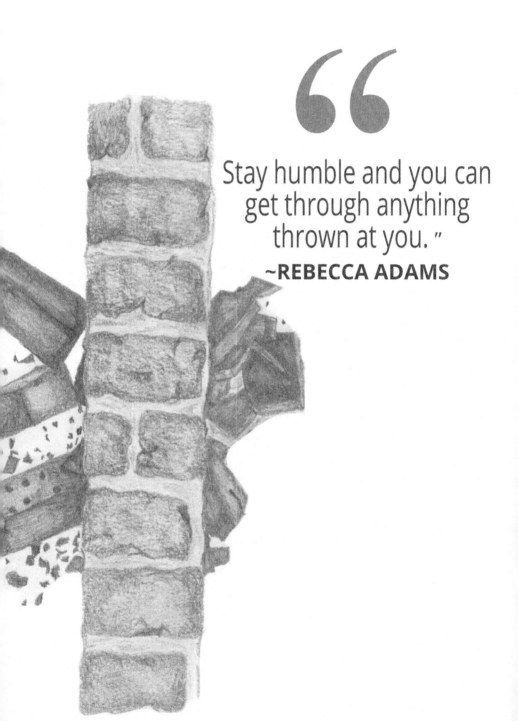

"Stay humble and you can get through anything thrown at you. "

~REBECCA ADAMS

There truly is ALWAYS A WAY! You just have to know it and believe it. Live it and go for it!

Your journey of life is and can be beautiful so strive to live a life full of abundance, love, joy, amazing opportunities, happiness, positivity and wonderful experiences so you can make beautiful memories and be surrounded by outstanding human beings.

You can do it! Have faith in you!

Remember – you're worth more than rubies and diamonds.

Rebecca Adams.x

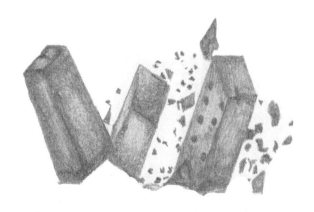

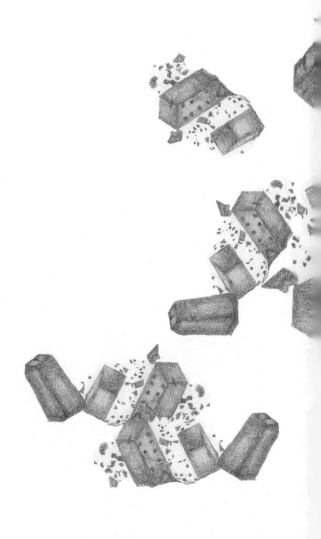
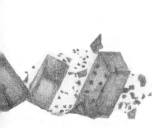

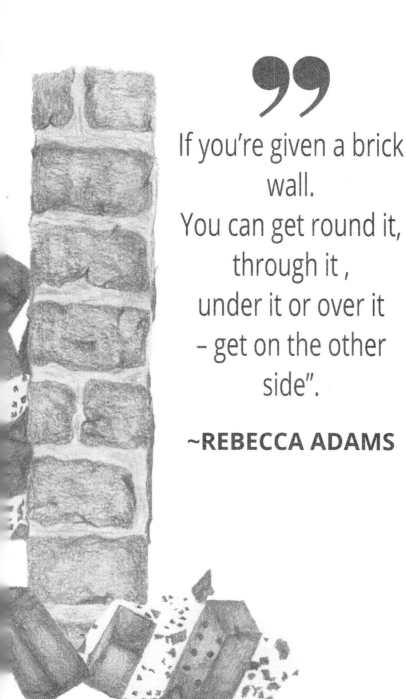

" If you're given a brick
wall.
You can get round it,
through it ,
under it or over it
- get on the other
side".

~REBECCA ADAMS

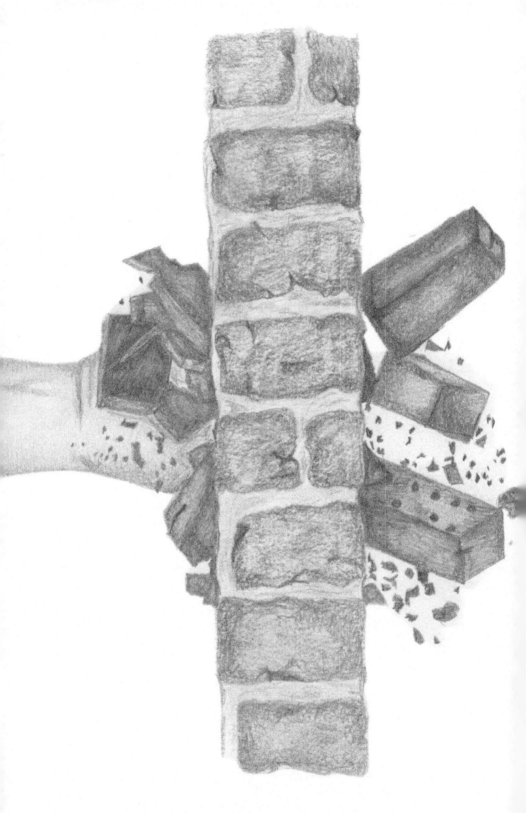

IN THAT SPLIT SECOND OUR LIVES CHANGED FOREVER

That scream kept me awake in the night for hours over a period of 6 months.

love to drive. I always have, ever since I got my driving licence. I love views, I love the open road and the scenery. It's absolute bliss to me. It is not about just getting from A to B - it's a whole wonderful and joyful experience. But everything changed one day in September 2013 when I was on the way home from Birmingham with my friends and team in my car.

We had just left the M4 motorway at Chippenham and were travelling back to drop C off at home. M wanted food so we stopped off and then said bye to C and were making our way back to my hometown.

The traffic lights were red, and we were third in a queue at the lights when they turned green but neither of the two cars in front of us moved. So, I presumed that the first driver had stalled the car and we were waiting for them to restart and move forward – not a problem at all.

There was a small car behind us, and we were all waiting. The first car started to move and so then did the second when all of a sudden, my friend S, who was sat in the back of the car, let out the most high-pitched scream I have ever heard in my life.

In that split second our lives changed forever....

The car behind us smashed into my car and moved us forward so we were through the lights. I hit my brakes so fast whilst the scream carried on. It was awful! My eyes were focused on not hitting the car in front of me, which did drive off unscathed from any of the accident.

I looked at my friend M, who was sat beside me in the front of the car with wide eyes and said "What the hell just happened? Are you okay?" and I then asked S too.

All of a sudden, a BMW appeared next to us. The front of the car was all smashed up and crumpled, together with the number plate half hanging off. The driver got out and so did the people in the car behind us. I looked at M and asked; "What do we do?". I had no idea – whether it was the shock or not I don't know but I had never been in an accident before so with the adrenalin pumping round, I just couldn't think straight.

We got out of the car and spoke to the people in the car behind. I spoke to the BMW driver who insisted because we were all walking that we were fine and not to phone the emergency services. He ripped his number plate off and threw it into his car. His excuse for the crash – "The lights were green!" Like, what?! Are you joking?! He wanted to leave the scene and so I told him he wasn't going anywhere without swapping details. He reluctantly did in the end, and he drove off!

We, however decided to phone the emergency services, and decided to wait at the fast-food restaurant opposite where the crash had happened. Whilst we were waiting, we asked around for witnesses and if the CCTV caught anything so we could give it to the police. S didn't feel well at all, so we took her into the restrooms. The fast-food restaurant gave us free drinks and food and they were absolutely amazing for us all that night. I wrote an amazing post on Facebook for them thanking them for their wonderful hospitality.

The police and ambulance arrived, and it wasn't until I informed them that they were missing the actual car that caused this entire thing because the driver had driven off – that they realised this was not as simple as two cars hitting each other. They were bewildered and shocked. We were all interviewed individually, and breath tests taken too, to make sure none of us were drinking. We were also checked over by the ambulance staff. The police then went off to the address given to us by the BMW driver. The entirety of the human beings that helped that night was astounding, and I thank each and every one of them.

> **They were bewildered and shocked.**

4 hours later I arrived home. It was only the next day that the pain and stiffness and the after-effects of the car crash started to take over my body. Oh wow! It was horrendous! Even though it was a Sunday I received a call about my car from the BMW driver's insurance company! Like what?! I was in complete shock. My pain was getting worse, and I was by myself with my children and they just wanted to sort money out! Wow! I remember thinking "They couldn't wait until Monday?!".

That night I couldn't sleep. Every time I closed my eyes the car crash happened again and again, and the scream kept me awake. I was in complete agony with my back and neck. I was in floods of tears!

I was absolutely exhausted when Monday morning arrived. My son got picked up to go to his special school, my daughter had to walk herself to school, and my beautiful and amazing Mum had arranged to come and stay for 6 days to help me out with the children. As she lived "up north" she couldn't travel down straight away. I phoned the doctors and explained what had happened and that I needed an appointment. The one thing that a lot of people were shocked about was that I still continued with the incentive I had set my business team. It was a spa day at a local hotel, and they thoroughly enjoyed it all. The ones of us in the crash were in so much pain that we didn't – not really. We could hardly walk.

> Anger took over me - this guy just smashed into us all in the queue at the lights and doesn't even know the ripple effect...

I couldn't move my neck, bend down to put my socks on and every step I took to walk around my house hurt. I couldn't even position myself in bed to sleep as the pain took over. I found it extremely difficult to get in and out of the shower and doing all the things we take for granted as able-bodied people. I felt every pain shoot through my body, and I was in complete tears.

Anger took over me - this guy just smashed into us all in the queue at the lights and doesn't even know the ripple effect that's taken place afterwards!

I was put on so much medication I went "do-lally" as I am small in height and build, they affected me a lot. I was referred to physiotherapy for my back and neck and told that because I couldn't move my neck, I was not allowed to drive at all. I couldn't anyway as my car had been written off and I won't ever forget the day that my silver car was towed away. I was in absolute tears seeing it on the back of the truck. I had worked and dreamed of having the car and it was taken from me, just like a click of the fingers. My Mum hugged me as I was crying, and we slowly went back into the house. That night I had work to do on my laptop, so Mum helped me out because I couldn't focus well, due to the medication I was on, but as the business didn't stop, I showed up and continued with the work that needed to be completed – namely congratulating my team on their work.

Every night the scream kept happening in my head from that night.

Every night I had no more than a few hours' sleep due to the amount of pain I was in.

Months of excruciating painful physio sessions followed, as Jo tried her best to get my back and neck to how they should be. But the one thing that I didn't count on was that my mindset had been knocked considerably, to the extent that I didn't want to get into a car - not any car! Like ever!

That was my brick wall. It was brick after brick rising up higher and higher.

So, my trips to the doctors and physio were fully of anxiety for me which included closing my eyes, deep breathing and lots of eating mints. "I didn't want to be in a piece of metal as that's not enough to shield me. A car can smash into the back of me at any time". Those thoughts right there, kept repeating in my head so much that I was referred to CBT sessions with a lovely lady named M.

Every session I was emotional and got upset because as a person I can switch anything around from any scenario at all but there was something different about this situation and I needed M to help me flick the switch and start to knock the brick walls down that were consuming me.

> **"**
> The bricks of the wall in front of you may have been put there by yourself, someone else or a situation you have witnessed or been part of...

She actively listened a lot, asked me questions, gave me tasks to do – which I am proud to say I did, even though many were uncomfortable and testing me, I accomplished them all and I didn't waiver, stop or refuse to do any of them. It was amazing for me.

The bricks of the wall in front of you may have been put there by yourself, someone else or a situation you have witnessed or been part of. Mine was the car accident. But the one thing I want you to acknowledge is that with the correct tools, people and support you can start to knock down those bricks one by one and start to rebuild your life again – no matter how long it takes. Go for the long game and go for a win-win.

In my case, as I lived down south, and my Mum lived "up north" in England I've always needed to drive long distance and I needed to be confident in the car again. Not everyone ends up in a car accident. I was and still am a really good driver and I was not to blame at all. These are the sentences that were repeated to me again and again whilst in CBT and also with having the physio sessions too, all of these amazing human beings helped me to rebuild my life – physically, emotionally and mentally too. I will always be grateful to them.

The brick wall that suddenly went up on that night started to collapse brick by brick as I took each day as it was and pushed myself that bit further. When I got behind the wheel of my new car I was upset. I just sat there for a short while in the car. The next step for me was to turn the engine on and sit there. Listen to the music playing and then go for a short drive round the block with someone in the car with me was the next step after that.

Each small step amounted to confidence building, even though I was conscious of always looking in the rear-view mirror more often that eventually dissipated, and I returned to the 'Rebecca driver' that people know and trust. It's the best feeling in the world.

And yes, I'm back to loving to drive all over the UK – even moreso, because I know how easy it is for things to change in the blink of an eye.

The scream eventually disappeared from my memory and a new mattress was bought to help with my back and neck.

Our lives changed forever from that night. We have all gone off in different directions but the one thing that remains is that our health comes first because we all need to look after our children and families.

My message to you, the reader, is that no matter if that brick wall is so high it's unbelievable, know that you are strong enough to knock those bricks down one by one in order to see the sunrise or sunset on the other side. So, with focus and determination you can conquer anything. Believe in yourself and go for it! You have nothing to lose and everything to gain. And, with your journey you may inspire others when sharing what you have been through.

> **I will always be grateful to the people who were part of that section of my life...**

I will always be grateful to the people who were part of that section of my life. It truly has transformed and shaped me as a person, and I've grown so much since that night. I am blessed to be surrounded by incredible human beings who believe in me as much as I believe in them and I submerse myself into my work and my calling each and every day to empower, inspire and motivate others, like yourself, to change their lives because life is so precious, and it can be over in the click of your fingers. Don't waste a moment.

Reach out, get the right support and know that you have the power within yourself to smash through your own brick wall.

DEDICATION.

I dedicate my chapter to my beautiful and inspirational Mum who took care of me during this time in my life. She dropped everything to come and help me and Mum, I am so grateful to you. x

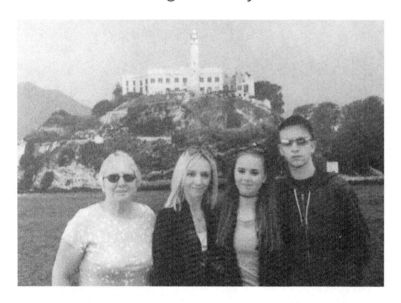

I also dedicate this chapter to M and S who were in the car that night and we were on that journey together. I am sending you both love. I also dedicate this chapter to J and M who helped me with physio and CBT. Gratitude. x

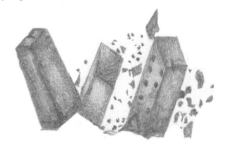

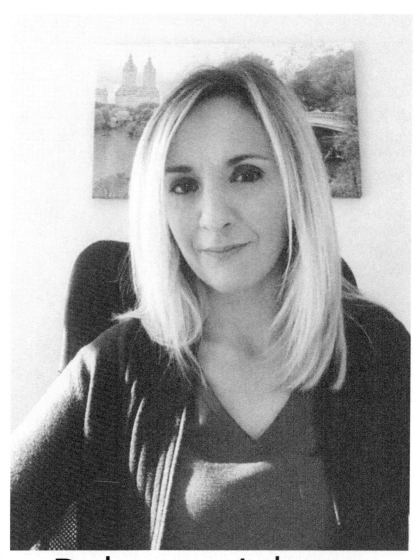

Rebecca Adams

Rebecca Adams

Rebecca Adams wears her heart on her sleeve and always flows in alignment through her life and business. She kicks ass at what she does, and she is focused on empowering as many people as possible to feel alive and live a phenomenal life through gaining control of their mindset and to be their true self. Her mission is to give more people the mindset, skillset and tools to gain more clarity, focus and confidence to master their life in all arenas, through aligning with their soul and doing the inner work needed.

Rebecca has been in business for over 18 years and she is all about empowering, inspiring and motivating people to uplevel, rise up, be a voice and to trust the process. She lives and breathes the Law of Attraction daily and is focused on giving as much value as possible to her audience.

She is the International Life, Business & Mindset Mastery Mentor™ for people who want to create personal and financial freedom. She is a Law of Attraction Practitioner, NLP Practitioner, Belief Clearing Practitioner, Author, Speaker, Motivator and Businesswoman. She builds websites, creates programs & helps people monetize their ideas.

Rebecca changes people's lives through her Transformational Digital Online Programs, High-end Private Bespoke Coaching & Mentoring. She also has an online membership club called Ignite Academy which is jampacked full of amazing content.

She is the Creative Director & Founder of the Empowerment Convention IGNITE Live Event which is a life-changing event with speakers, a gala dinner and entertainment, held annually in the Roman City of Bath, UK.
Rebecca is an award-winning entrepreneur, #1 International best-selling co-author, and masters in mindset. Unlike every other personal development expert, she focuses on aligning every area of your life so that you can take control and have everything you desire.

She is a Mum to 2 amazing incredible human beings, a Special Needs Mum, a UK Army Veteran and she lives in the UK. She loves to travel, read, listen to music, take photographs, watch movies and make endless memories. She is a dedicated daughter to her inspirational Mum Carole.

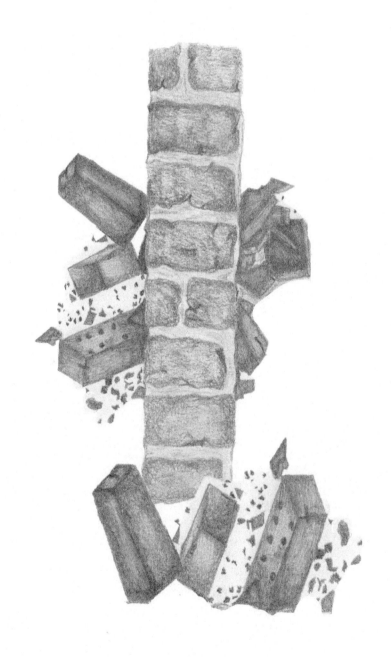

Rebecca was nominated for the 2019 Boots Wellness Warrior of the Year Award and also the 2019 Businesswoman of the Year Award.
She has also been nominated for 2 awards in the DIGITAL WOMEN AWARDS 2021.

WEB LINKS:
Website: https://www.rebeccaadamsbiz.com
Business Facebook Page: https://www.facebook.com/rebeccaadams187
Personal Facebook Wall: https://www.facebook.com/rebecca.adams.39108/
Online Digital Course Website: http://racourses.thinkific.com/
Linktree: https://linktr.ee/rebeccaadams187
Instagram: https://www.instagram.com/rebeccaadams187
Pinterest: https://www.pinterest.com/rebeccaadams187
Clubhouse: @rebeccaadams187

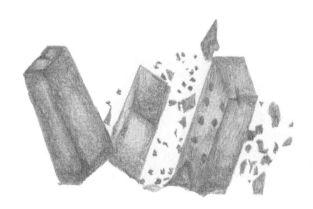

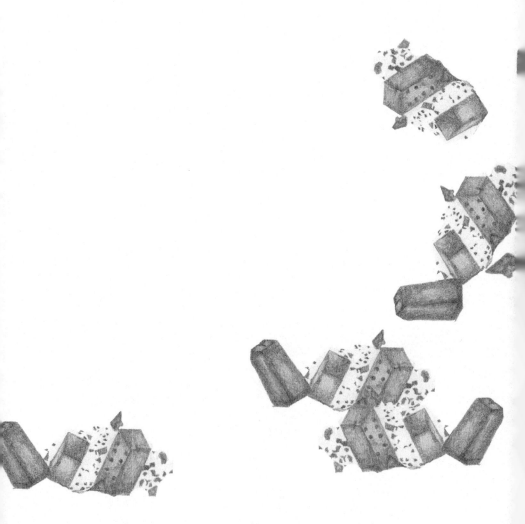

"

Never give up hope.
Keep positive and Stay
Strong"

~CAROLE ARNOLD

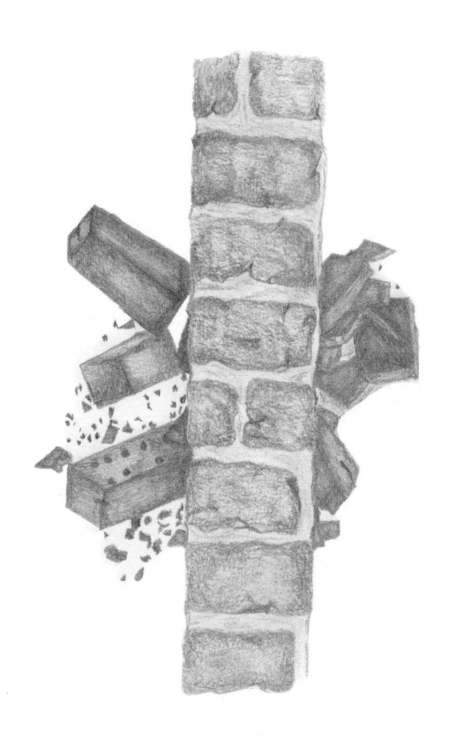

"The Big C"

CAROLE ARNOLD

Those are 3 little words people dread hearing...

The fear sets in when you hear this and then it starts to play havoc with your mind. The questions creep in – "Why me?" "What have I been doing that I've got this?" "Have I been living the wrong lifestyle or eating the wrong foods?".

Given this diagnosis is not necessarily a death sentence anymore. Lots of research has been done and great strides have been made in eradicating some cancers. The one thing I can tell you (as someone who has had, and still has, cancer (which I will go into detail further along) is – "Never give up hope. Keep positive and Stay Strong".

My cancer journey started in late 2017, when I noticed I was losing weight, my appetite had decreased, and I was a lot more tired than usual. I knew this wasn't normal (as an ex-nurse of over 23+ years) so I went to my GP who then arranged for me to have a CT scan which showed a mass on the left side of my abdomen. A biopsy, in the new year of 2018, confirmed Non-Hodgkins Lymphoma.

This shocked me even though I had an inkling that it was something serious. "Oh well", I thought, "let's get this sorted, I can beat this". So, I was admitted to hospital a week later for my first course of chemotherapy. All went well with no reaction (thankfully) and so I had to attend the oncology suite every three weeks for regular chemotherapy.

And guess what? My hair fell out!!

> "Oh well",
> I thought,
> "let's get this sorted,
> I can beat this"

I mean all of it fell out, apart from my eyebrows and eyelashes. To this day, I still have none on my legs or under my arms (suppose it saves on buying razor's anyway!). Luckily, there is a wig service at the hospital, and you are allowed one wig free of charge and I did have a lovely one made for me (now in a box in a cupboard).

Just after course 5, I contracted Neutropenic Sepsis which is a serious condition in itself, and I was transferred to hospital for intense intravenous antibiotics and fluids. I had caught this sepsis in time and was discharged 4 days later. I had to also have 6 days of injections to increase my immune system.

At the same time that this was going on I attended my local Breast Unit for a usual mammogram. I was called back into the Unit 2 weeks later for an ultrasound as something looked suspicious on the mammogram. A core biopsy was done which showed I had a Grade 1 cancer, and a 'marker' was inserted to see the site of the cancer.

I was very emotional. "Here we go again!! Most people get cancer once but oh no not me I had to have it twice". I would have to wait before they operated because I was going to undergo 15 sessions of radiology on the Lymphoma first.

I had to travel to another out-of-town hospital. The NHS Transport service were very good at getting me there as I didn't have a clue of where it was. I went 5 days a week for 3 weeks and I remember having radiotherapy actually on my birthday. I can certainly think of better ways to spend your birthday! The radiology staff were absolutely lovely and even gave me a birthday cake on the day. The results on this course of chemotherapy and radiotherapy did the trick with the Lymphoma.

> ""
> I remember having radiotherapy actually on my birthday.
> I can certainly think of better ways to spend your birthday!

 "Right," I thought, "one down - one to go. Keep positive and let's get on with this".

A fortnight later, in October, I had my pre-op ready for my operation a month later. They gave me a radioactive sentinel lymph node injection prior to the operation the day after. A blue dye was administered, (which gave me a blue breast for weeks), to the cancer and some surrounding tissue. Plus, lymph nodes in my armpit were removed under general anaesthetic. I healed well with no infection.

CAROLE ARNOLD

Two weeks later I was seen in clinic and given the "all clear". They had removed the cancer successfully and there hadn't been any spread to the lymph nodes. Phew, what a relief it was to hear that. "Two down - Now to get on with my life".

How wrong was I.

Nine months later, in June 2019, I was diagnosed with Grade 4 colorectal cancer. "Not again", I thought. The old adage did creep in at this stage and I did think; "Why me?" But there was no use wallowing in self-pity. I had to get on with it and beat this disease one more time.

> **Nine months later, in June 2019, I was diagnosed with Grade 4 colorectal cancer.**

I wasn't going to have my operation until November of 2019, so I took myself off to Las Vegas in the USA in August, (I didn't mind going on my own) and it's where I had a brilliant time exploring the Grand Canyon, enjoying a Cirque du Soleil show at the MGM Grand, having a helicopter ride over the Strip at night, etc.

Operation day came and went, and when the consultant came to see me, he told me he had removed all the cancer, a few lymph nodes and half of my bowel. "Good", I thought – "another one got rid of. Now to get on with my life again".

I organised a trip to Bali in Indonesia with my sister Sue. I love to travel as there's so much of the world to see and make memories. We had a truly incredible time and as soon as I returned, I had my follow up CT scan which is routine in these cancer cases. I was astonished to hear that I also had to have an MRI scan. This showed up liver metastasis and apparently I had four of these 'hotspots' on my liver. I thought to myself "When is this ever going to end?".

Chemotherapy started again which had to be changed to a different regime as I was too ill on the first regime. The second different regime was even worse, and this stopped after 3 treatments. My newly grown hair was lost again!! It was a good job that I still had my wig (which is now, again, sitting unused in a box)!

I ended up in hospital again this time with bi-lateral pulmonary embolisms (blood clots in both lungs). I was discharged on blood thinning injections (which I have now been told I'm on for ever and a day) and which make me feel like a pin cushion as I have to inject into my stomach twice a day. (This has since been changed to oral tablets, so it is much better and obviously less painful).

> *I ended up in hospital again this time with bi-lateral pulmonary embolisms (blood clots in both lungs).*

This was a time when I became at my lowest point and I broke down in my kitchen and sobbed my heart out. I just didn't know how much more I could take. Having one cancer and beating it is enough for anyone, but this was number four! It just didn't seem fair. Then I gave myself a good talking to, dusted myself down and decided to stay strong and stay positive. I have always been a fighter from being a small child so I sure as hell wasn't going to give in now!!

I started a new course of chemotherapy which is in tablet form only and which I can take at home, and which seems to suit me. I thought that this would be on-going and end with a cure or a slowing down of the disease. However, this is not happening now as a recent CT scan has shown the liver "hotspots" are not improving and so all chemotherapy treatment has been stopped.

Whatever course my body decides to take on this, I will enjoy life as best I can. As the group "Journey" used in one of their powerful title songs, "Don't Stop Believing" - and I won't.

So, I am not giving up hope and never will, and I am staying positive. Hope is being able to see that there is light despite all of the darkness, and everything is a fresh beginning. If you put your mind to it, you can and will achieve anything as life is precious and is for living.

I know my prognosis, but I still have lots to do and go for whilst on this planet and I'm making sure I do.

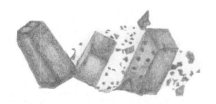

DEDICATION

I should like to dedicate this story to my wonderful daughter Becci, who has kept me positive throughout and sat with me through hours of treatment and who has been my rock.

Love you girl. (2x heart emoji's)

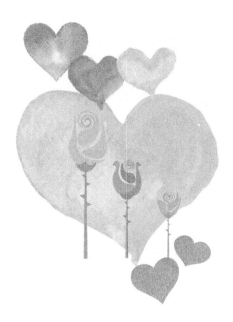

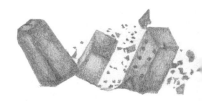

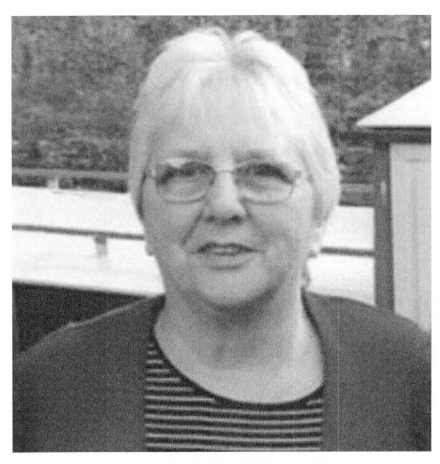

Carole Arnold

Carole Arnold

Carole is a retired Registered General Nurse (RGN) of 23yrs, of which she is very proud of. She is a Mum, wife, sister and she also is devoted to her little dog Charlie.

Carole absolutely loves to travel and has been to so many countries she has lost track! She has lots of photos and amazing memories from all the places she has visited as a solo traveller, as well as with her sister Sue, daughter Rebecca and husband Bill.

Over the years she has been an incredible mentor within her career and is an inspirational role model to many. She loves to laugh, watch comedies and crime programs.

Social Media Link:

Facebook: www.facebook.com/carole.arnold.9

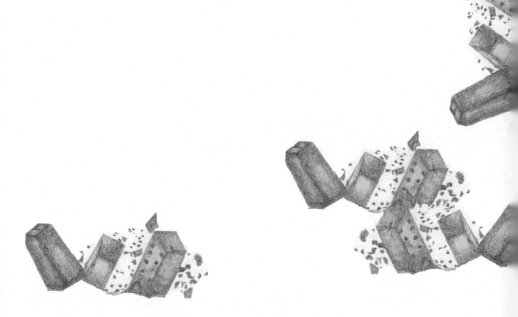

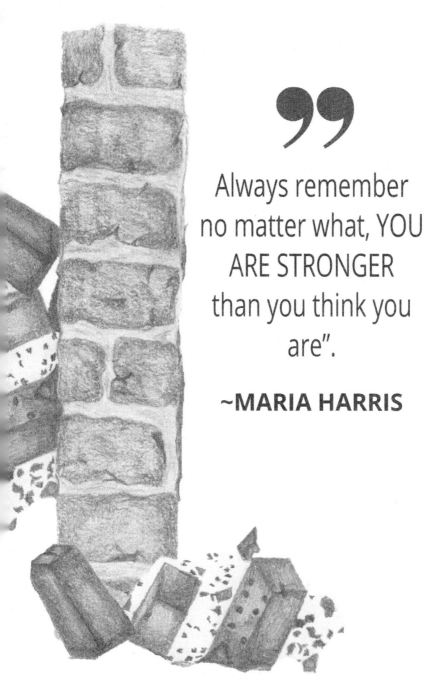

Always remember
no matter what, YOU
ARE STRONGER
than you think you
are".

~MARIA HARRIS

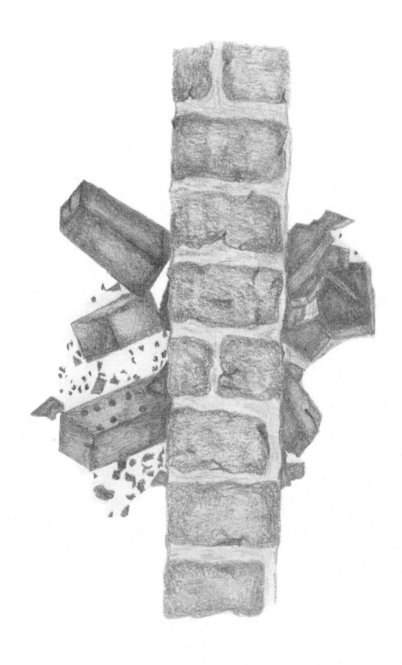

When a Family holiday takes an unexpected turn!

Let me start by taking you back to 2015.
As September was fast approaching,
(it's always a bad month as I lost my dad in September 2011)
my mum and I always went on holiday for the
anniversary, as it always felt right.

This year was no different, so we booked to go away for 2 weeks for dads' anniversary and this year we took my friend with us too. We set off on our family holiday full of joy and happiness and couldn't wait to get to our favourite little bar for the lasagne and garlic bread - a meal both my mum and I loved.

Arriving in Gran Canaria, we felt like we were home and were ready to enjoy our holiday, make more memories and catch up with friends we had made over there. Me and my mum used to go every year for the last 7 years, so we'd made some really great friends with the locals. We arrived at our hotel and were given apartment 126. We dropped our bags off and set off for our meal we had been waiting for. It was just as we remembered and was definitely well worth the wait. After we had eaten, we went and got a few bits from the supermarket to take back to the room.

The first week was really enjoyable showing my friend around the local areas, going for a swim, chilling and relaxing on the sea front, shopping and catching up with our friends. On the Sunday morning we went down to the seafront for breakfast where we could look out across the sea and around the island. We were sat eating breakfast just having a general chat and my mum looks at me and says "Ri, I'm not coming home with you", to which my reply was "yes you are mum what are you on about?"

What I wasn't prepared for was her response to what I had said. She came out with "I'm coming home in a box". Shocked and taken off guard at this point was a complete understatement. I looked at my mum and said, "don't be silly mum you're coming home with us". Mum changed the subject, and we went on with our day.

> " I'm coming home in a box".
> Shocked and taken off guard at this point was a complete understatement...

My head being completely baffled by what my mum had said, and it had kind of thrown me off guard, but I was determined to enjoy the holiday. We had been trying to track a friend down on the island, who had moved jobs so that evening we went for a little wander to see if we could find our friend. We found the bar they were working in, but mum was feeling tired, so we got a taxi back to the apartment and sat on our balcony playing cards and having a drink.

Monday morning arrived and my mum woke up feeling a bit under the weather and not too good, so we spent most of the day on the balcony whilst my mum slept, and she joined us every now and then. We managed to take mum out that evening for some tea and went straight back to the hotel room. Mum said she was happy for me and my friend to go down to the bar and see if we could find our friend and have a catch up at the local drag cabaret bar.

My friend and I went down to the local bar and found our friend and so, we stayed to watch the show and had a nice evening chilling, watching our friend in action of course with a few drinks. We left the bar and headed back to the hotel and to check in on my mum. When we got back my mum was still awake and waiting for us to get back. We sat, had a chat then we all went to bed.

Tuesday morning, we all woke up and mum still wasn't right, full of cold, not wanting to eat - only drink fluids, which, with her diabetes, wasn't great. So, we had another day chilling out and I took mum to the hotel bar and got her something to eat and drink and told her she needed to try and eat something. Mum eventually had her lunch. We were just casually sat there, and mum said, "Ri what's sitting on the bin?" I turned round, had a look but there wasn't anything there. So, I replied "there's nothing there, you must be seeing things" but mum was adamant that there was something there. We went back to our room and sat out on the balcony. Mum was staring into space and looked at me, "Ri who is that stood over there watching us?"

Again, I looked and was shocked as no one was there. So, I told mum there was nothing there. She then said, "I thought you could see the other side Ri". I replied, "I can but not all the time mum I'm not that type of person". Mum went off for a nap and me and my friend popped down to the supermarket. Whilst we were there, I remember having a conversation with my friend saying I was worried, as it seemed mum was hallucinating, but her sugar levels were okay as I had been keeping an eye on them. My friend agreed with me that it was weird. We went back to the room and again mum still wasn't feeling great, so we had our meal in the room. Mum didn't feel up to going out and was coughing really badly again but told me and my friend to go out. My friend and I got ready and headed back down into town. I said I wanted to try and see if I could get mum some tablets from the doctor or pharmacist as I wasn't sure what I could give her because of her medication.

MARIA HARRIS

Although I can speak some Spanish it was really difficult to try and explain what medicine my mum was taking. We went off to the bar and again had a good night. We went back to our room and mum was already asleep. That night I was woken up by mum going through the wardrobe saying she needed to find her uniform as she had to go work. She was pulling all the clothes out trying to find a uniform that wasn't there. I gave her some paracetamol and told her to get some sleep and she'd feel better in the morning.

Wednesday morning, we all woke up and headed down to the seafront for some breakfast, as I know my mum liked the breakfast down there and thought it would be a good way to get her to eat. Afterwards we headed back to the hotel pool. At this point mum still was not right at all so I phoned the UK and got her doctor to ring me with some advice as I was growing more concerned about my mum as she was still seeing things and not really making much sense.

The doctors rang me back quickly and agreed to change her medication round a bit and advised me to get her to have a sleep. So, we went back to our apartment and I gave mum her medication and told her to have a nap. She woke up and said she was feeling better and wanted to come out with us to see our friend. So, we got a taxi to town, got burgers and fries and went to the bar. We had a lovely evening with mum having a few drinks, giggles etc and then headed back to the hotel about 2am.

Into Thursday – A DAY I'LL NEVER FORGET FOR THE REST OF MY LIFE – Our family holiday went devastatingly wrong!

We all went to sleep after a good evening out. Around 9am I got woken up by my mum grabbing my arm in her sleep or what I thought was sleep. I shrugged her off and turned over and went back to sleep.

I woke around 10.30am, went and made a coffee and sat outside on the balcony where my friend joined me. I kept checking on mum as thought it was strange, she was not awake yet. My friend and I took it in turns to go and check on her. About 11am we heard a random noise from the bedroom, so we went in to check on mum. On entering the room, I noticed my mum's face had gone blue! You can imagine the thoughts and panic running through my head at this point. Imagine being in a hotel in a foreign country, no other family with you and seeing your mum laying there all blue.

I jumped onto the bed and shook my mum, shouted at her, tapped her across the face (as I initially thought she'd gone into a diabetic coma). She wasn't responding at all, so I grabbed the phone and called the emergency services who hung up on me as they didn't understand me. As you can imagine the horror, panic and adrenaline all hitting me at once, now what do I do...?

I ran to a neighbour's apartment to get help and the husband helped me with my mum checking for a pulse whilst his wife rang reception to get an ambulance. Neither of us could find a pulse and I just cried and screamed.

> ❞
> As you can imagine the horror, panic and adrenaline all hitting me at once, now what do I do....?

The neighbours then advised me to ring the travel agency to get advice. Within 30 minutes the manager was sat with me on our balcony and was guiding me through the process and what to do. He advised me to get straight onto the insurance company so plans can be arranged and sorted for mum and for our flight home.

The ambulance crew then arrived who also could not find a pulse but in Spain the protocols are completely different to in the UK. They had to then call the police who came out and checked mum and they had to call the judge and doctor to come out. The ambulance crew left as the police arrived.

The police removed mine and my friend's passports and from that point, we weren't allowed to enter the room and we always being watched. If we needed anything we had to be escorted at all times and had to stay outside on the balcony in the burning hot sun with next to no shade.

> Once the judge arrived, he officially declared mum had passed away...

The doctor arrived and by this point we knew mum had died.

He took details from my friend and I about the events leading up to that day including mum's health, etc. Once the judge arrived, he officially declared mum had passed away and arranged for mum to be collected and taken to the morgue.

By this point it was 3.45pm and this had been going on since 11am. As our room was on the opposite side of the complex, mum had to be wheeled out through the hotel and around the pool! This was by no means the hardest part, as all other holiday makers could then see mum being wheeled away in a body bag.

Now, you would have thought that was the most dramatic part...... but no it got worse.

Once the insurance company had taken all the information, they advised they would get their end rolling and let me know if the claim was accepted and what the next steps were. Well, I then received a phone call to tell me the claim had not been accepted and I would be liable to pay £9,000 to get my mum home.

I questioned as to why it wasn't accepted, and they advised that some of my mum's health conditions were not mentioned within the policy. I set the policies up, so I know all her health conditions were on there. I advised the person of this and told them to recheck the policy and to come back to me.

By this point I'd just lost my mum in Gran Canaria, and now being told I had to pay to get her home, my emotions were going mad, and I didn't know what to do, where to go or what to say. After 30 minutes they rang me back and said they'd found the other health conditions as it had gone into a different screen, as there were quite a few listed. The claim was now accepted, and they guided me through the process on what was next.
By this point I was sunburnt, hot, bothered, upset, worried and I just wanted a drink to calm my nerves. So, my friend and I went to the hotel bar and got a couple of brandy's to help with the last few painful hours. The hotel was amazing as they didn't charge us for our drinks and people were lovely, coming across to us and offering their help and support. We spoke to the travel rep who came and sat with us for another drink and to explain to me I had to go to court the next morning to put my statement in and at that point we would get our passports back, which I was glad about, as we just wanted to go home.

We went back to the room.......although I couldn't face being in there. We got changed and went out to the drag bar to explain to our friend what had happened. Again, the bar was amazing as they didn't charge us for many of our drinks throughout the evening and even played a few of our favourite acts to help us get through this difficult time. We headed back to the hotel around 4am and set about trying to get some sleep. Yeah, that just wasn't happening!

Friday morning came - the day before we were due to fly home. The day I had to go to court to explain what had happened. My nerves were through the roof to say the least. A travel rep met us outside to help guide me through the process and help with any translations that were needed. Once this was done, we headed back to the hotel for some lunch, with our passports that had been handed back.

MARIA HARRIS

The insurance company rang me to say I had to get the paper-work from reception with mum's death certificate before I was allowed to fly home and that they should be at reception by 5pm. We were flying home the next day and being collected at 4.05pm to be taken to the airport to come home. 5pm came and went and still no paperwork was dropped off to us. I rang the insurance again and they said to let them know if nothing had been received by midday on Saturday.

Onto Saturday morning and I still hadn't got much sleep and still no paperwork! So, I rang the insurance company to ask If I was allowed to fly home or what did I need to do. They said they'd find out and let me know.

Panic set in...... we were being picked up at 4.05pm and it was now 3pm, and I still hadn't heard a thing, so I rang them back and said, "I have an hour before my transfer. What is going on as I still have no paperwork?" At 3.30pm they rang me back and advised I could fly home and that the paperwork would be sent back with my mum. That gave me 30mins to pack up and make it to reception.

Back at the airport and I then had the task of trying to explain why I had 3 people's luggage and only two people. This was a nightmare and just another hurdle to get around. Finally, we got it sorted and headed to the gate to board the plane home. Once we had boarded the plane it was weird to have an empty seat and that set all emotions going again and I was in tears sat on the plane knowing mum was being left there on her own. Then to make matters worse, they had already sold my mum's seat, so I had a stranger sat next to me on the plane, again how I handled that for 4 hours on the way home I'll never know.
Once home I was greeted by my friends and I just broke down completely and didn't know what to do, as I then had funeral arrangements, getting mum home and everything else to do, all on my own. I am an only child and now an orphan. I didn't know what I was going to do.

If I was to give anyone any advice at all it would be to PLEASE, PLEASE, PLEASE, always get travel insurance. I don't care if you're going away for 3 days or 3 weeks - always make sure you have travel insurance and every tiny detail of medical history is listed, even the small things you think that don't matter. TRUST ME - they matter when something does happen.

And always remember no matter what, YOU ARE STRONGER than you think you are.

You can overcome every hurdle that is put in front of you.
I did not believe I was strong enough and when you go through something like this your strength will get you through. I certainly am strong, and it is an experience I will never ever forget.
Always cherish the time you have with your loved ones and your friends. I know I do.

DEDICATION
This chapter is dedicated to my daughter Ruby-Leigh who never got to meet her grandparents.
Also, to Ashley, for being by my side throughout this journey and still being there now.

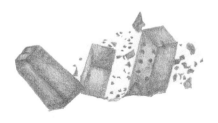

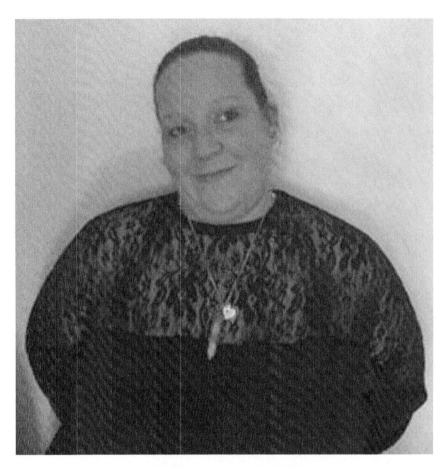

Maria Harris

Maria Harris

Maria is a single mum to daughter Ruby-Leigh. She lives in Swansea in Wales, although she grew up in Wiltshire. She enjoys listening to music and watching films in her spare time. She enjoys spending quality time with her daughter and friends.

In 2021 she embarked on a new journey in Wales and starting her own Business to work from home. She started Little Ruby's Treats, which is a printing, sweet hampers and hampers business. The business is slowly growing, and she is hoping to keep expanding the business in new ways as the business grows.

Social Links:
Website: www.littlerubystreats.co.uk
Personal Facebook: https://www.facebook.com/Shortie69/
Business Facebook: https://www.facebook.com/groups/lrtreats
Instagram: https://www.instagram.com/treatslittlerubys/
Linktree: https://linktr.ee/Littlerubystreats

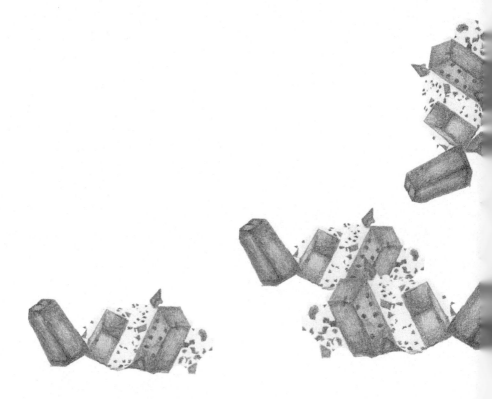

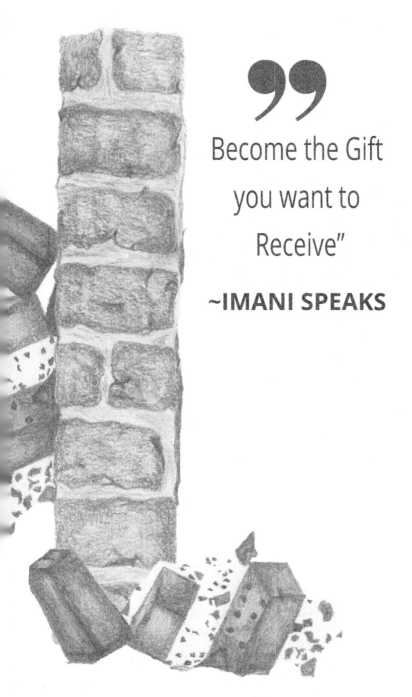

Become the Gift
you want to
Receive"

~IMANI SPEAKS

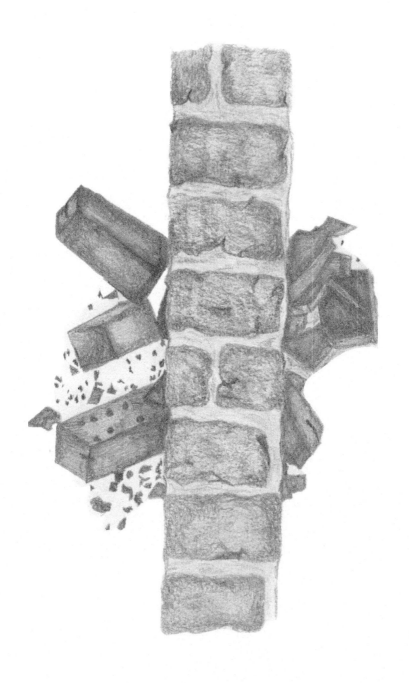

The EVER Changing You
FALL, RISE & SHINE

Beginning of the New Year

It was the New Year, and Faye had set aside some time to do some goal setting for the year ahead. She picked up her pen to write in her gratitude journal, but the words were not flowing through her. Faye had some successes last year but was also a little disappointed. She knew that she could have achieved much more. Faye was feeling a little restless not as focused as she needed to be for the occasion.

The month was fresh and new, but Faye was not feeling very motivated. She knew that she had much to be grateful for - her family, friends and the fact that she was in good health. She needed to unleash her superpowers of gratitude, love, courage and resourcefulness.

Let this year be about bringing out the true YOU,
It is about who you're BE-ING not what you do

From caterpillar to BUTTERFLY
Spread your wings and fly

Don't let nothing stop your flight
Set your sight on the highest height

IMANI SPEAKS

RE-MEMBER who you really are
Celebrities are nice, but you are the real STAR

Shine your light as bright as can be
Reveal your authenticity

Fly like the beautiful butterfly you truly are
Don't let nothing stop you from reaching your STAR

Without the caterpillar there'd be no butterfly
Without the metamorphosis they'd be no wings for you to fly

THE BUS RIDE OF HER LIFE

As she began to write in her journal, she found herself reflecting on the long-ago past. She remembers the vague, hazy memory of when she was only five years old and had fallen under a moving bus. She remembers her grandmother pleading with the bus conductor to stop the bus. Miraculously Little Faye was unhurt, no scars, no injuries.

GRATITUDE IS A SUPERPOWER

Faye could feel the superpower of gratitude flowing through her heart. She was thankful to have another day to do better than the day before. She was grateful for the New Year, the new day and all the beautiful experiences that would come her way.
Faye took several deep breaths, and more memories from the past started to flood her mind.

NO MORE ICE CREAM ON SUNDAYS

Faye and Patricia were best friends and looked forward to meeting up at Sunday school. The lady preaching on the rostrum that day was a guest preacher from America. She had chosen a rather strange topic as her sermon 'Death in the Pot?'. Faye and Patricia looked at each other, bemused, not quite sure what this lady preacher was saying. They had more important things on their mind like checking the clock, wondering when the church service would be over so that they could go and get their favourite ice-cream from the ice-cream van across the road.

The lady preacher continued to preach about 'Death in the Pot', and Patricia and Faye kept looking at the clock. Finally, the lady preacher finished her sermon, and the congregation prayed, and the service was over. Everyone gathered outside the courtyard of the church, meeting and greeting each other.

They had been dreaming of the moment when they could eat their ice-cream. The girls had been patient for so long, listening to that long sermon. It was a warm summer's day; it seemed like they had been in church for the longest time.

Faye and Patricia knew that they deserved to have their favourite ice-cream, so with coins in hand, they beamed with excitement and off they went.

Faye and Patricia quickly rushed outside; the moment they'd both been waiting for had finally arrived. They could see the ice-cream van from across the road.

They stood at the curb looked left and right, and left again, (as they had been taught to do) and started to cross the road. Suddenly, from out of nowhere, there was a loud bang, and a deafening silence and then chaos. Faye was numb; she could not move; she stared down at the ground where her best friend Patricia lay unconscious, her coins scattered on the ground beside her. Faye could not believe what had happened.

> **Suddenly, from out of nowhere, there was a loud bang, and a deafening silence and then chaos...**

Why had this happened to Patricia, thought Faye. Why were we being punished? Was it because we wanted ice-cream and were not paying attention to the preaching? Had the lady preacher caused this to happen – with her death in the pot message? We were just two little girls, how could God let this happen. Patricia was a good little girl. She did not hurt anyone; she said her prayers, loved her family; she was a good friend.

IMANI SPEAKS

A few moments ago, they were two happy giggling ten-year-olds looking forward to eating their favourite ice-cream. Now everything had changed - forever.

The ambulance arrived and took Patricia and her mother to the hospital. Would Patricia survive? No-one had the answers. They all had to wait to find out. Later that evening, Faye's mum received the call that Patricia did not make it. She was gone - just like that. Faye was devastated that she had not been able to say goodbye to her best friend. Weeks after the funeral, Faye was numb, quiet and still in shock, unable to accept what had happened.

> **They were two happy giggling ten-year-olds looking forward to eating their favourite ice-cream...**

Patricia was the youngest girl of three children; she was the only girl in her family. Patricia was their little angel, and now she was gone. She was a great friend; she was funny, kind and always cheerful. She was the kind of person who brought out the best in others. She was a beautiful soul who made other children feel good when she was around.

Over the weeks, months and years since Patricia's death, Faye felt uncomfortable even guilty having survived. Seeing the empty seat where Patricia used to sit during Sunday school, would bring back memories of that day.

Patricia's mum would always stare at Faye, with sad eyes without a smile; lost in her thoughts. It made Faye feel uneasy. This broken-hearted mother said nothing, but her eyes said everything. Faye felt sad for Patricia's mum; she felt awful. Faye wondered why God had allowed her to live - yet allowed Patricia to die. Patricia's death had also stolen her mother's smile.

Growing up as a child in church, Faye attended many weddings, christenings and funerals. However, no other death or funeral (at that time) impacted Faye like her best friend's untimely death.

REVIEWING THE PAST, IN THE PRESENT MOMENT
Faye had mixed feelings about these memories thinking how poignant they were. She realised that for most of her life, she had been playing small. At times, Faye would hide away or sabotage her goals, not allowing herself to progress. Was she playing small in life because of the loss of her best friend all those years ago? Did she believe, deep down inside, that she did not deserve to win in the game of life?

Faye reflected on how she had been walking through life apologizing for taking up space in the world. She was playing small and being a people-pleaser, not feeling like she fit in or belonged anywhere. Faye found it challenging to immerse herself in the game of life. She was always worrying about what others thought about her. Faye knew that things had to change; she knew how to change it. She would succeed and then sabotage her way back to square one. Faye had successes in her life, but she would not allow herself to play full out and give one hundred percent, she would always find a way to hold herself back. Faye started to write in her journal, affirmations on health and wellbeing which brought up memories of her health scare 21 years ago.

IN SICKNESS & IN HEALTH
'If You do not change your lifestyle, you will not live to see your next birthday.'

Those words from her doctor hit like a ton of bricks and was a real wake up call. Faye had gone to see her doctor for a check-up. She was not feeling well at all for some time. Faye was so sick that it started to affect her work attendance.

She knew that she could not carry on like this. She was in her mid-thirties at the time, only 5' 3" but weighing in at 14 stones, wearing size 22 clothing. When she first started the job, she was wearing size 10-12 clothing and weighing around 9.7 stones and had bags of energy.

IMANI SPEAKS

Her doctor wanted to prescribe a whole host of pills and potions, but Faye decided against it. She was determined to get her health back on track by adopting a healthy lifestyle that she would design. She had used her inner genius to change other areas of her life; now, she would use that same power to win back her health.

Faye had her work cut out for her; she was diagnosed with raging blood sugars, obesity, IBS, nervous indigestion and high blood pressure. Her energy was low, and she was in excruciating pain, particularly when she ate certain foods.

A lot was going on in Faye's life at that time, besides holding down two jobs; she was also working on starting a business. She had recently gone through a difficult divorce. She had neglected her health, was eating on the go (eating carelessly and unconsciously) and doing hardly any exercise. It did not help that her job was sedentary and that the chef's creations were so delicious, and to make matters worse, the portions were enormous. It seemed that the less active Faye was, the more she wanted to eat.

She would wake up in excruciating pain and have to ring in sick yet again for maybe the second time that week. She had to give up her locum work for a while but miraculously was still able to hold on to her main job. These painful episodes occurred over several months.

Faye realised that her presenting ailments were not the cause of her ill health, but were symptoms of something underlying. She had to get to the root of the problem. Faye realised that she had not been practising self-love and good self-care. She was neglecting the fact that she was a human being and not a human-Doing. Faye was doing too much and not relaxing into her Beingness. She was not conscious of what she was consuming spiritually, mentally, emotionally. All these stresses had manifested in her body as health challenges.

Faye knew that she had to rid herself of the excess stress. She needed to feel comfortable saying no, instead of being a people-pleaser and practice the art of being in her body through meditation. She also knew that she had to heal and let go of the past.

As Faye came out of her thoughts and back into the present day, she realised how far she had come. However, she knew that she still had a long way to go. She decided to do some more breath work, which always centres her and brings her back to the present moment!

PREPARING TO MEET THE FUTURE SELF

We are forever changing always moving towards becoming our future self.
A new year, a new month, a new day - a new Who? We are always moving towards our true self or away from our true self in every given moment – we get to choose!

> ❞
> We attract
> what we fear,
> love or hate...

The lyrics in the song asks the question,
Do you know where you're going to, do you like the things that life is showing you – where are you going to, do you know?'

We attract what we fear, love or hate. The emotion that is the strongest will attract the people around us, the circumstances we experience and who we are becoming. Life is always showing us the physical equivalent of our deepest beliefs, thoughts and emotions.

If we do not like what is showing up in our external life, the good news is that we can change it on the inside. The root cause is always the belief, followed by our thoughts and emotions.

At her next doctor's appointment, she got the all-clear. She was well, fit and back at work. That was twenty-one years ago and twenty-one more birthdays.

IMANI SPEAKS

Back to the Present Moment - Preparing to Meet the Future Self
Faye thought about how she had overcome so much in her past; she realised that she could no longer afford to play small and give up on herself. She had not seriously set any goals for a few years; she had allowed life to creep up on her.

Yes, Faye knew that she was getting older, but she had come to realise that whilst she was still breathing, she was still in the game of life, which meant that there is still time to make things happen.

The year was still new, and she still had time to use her gifts, abilities and talents to make a difference both in her life and in the life of others.

Faye knows that she cannot change the world, but knows that she can change her inner world, which will change how she shows up in the outer world. The Soul's journey is all about un-covering the ever-changing self, that is where the real work lies.

Have courage to be you
You are your own guru

You are the leader of your life
Unveil your true self with pride

Let your inner lion conquer
Your fears and make you stronger

Giving birth to your dreams
May sometimes seem surreal

But if you believe in yourself
You will find your inner wealth

Awaken the sleeping giant within
Don't allow your inner light to dim

Know that anything is possible
Because you are phenomenal

REVIEWING ACCOMPLISHMENTS AT THE END OF THE YEAR

It is December 31st, and Faye is preparing for the year ahead. She looks back and realises that she has achieved many of the goals that she set herself at the beginning of the year. She is looking forward to all that the new year has to offer. It was not an easy year, but it was a good year. She was able to remain conscious, focused and centred.

Faye allowed her inner genius to take charge, and she obeyed and took action. It was not easy for her to conquer her fears, and it was not easy for her to pick herself up after failures and begin again. Overcoming our fears and failures strengthens us and allows us to grow to the next level of our true authentic self.

Faye welcomes the ever-changing version of herself. Knowing that she will never be perfect, but accepting that she will always be the best person she can be at the time. She is ready to say goodbye to the old programming and old worn-out thinking patterns. She is exchanging old disempowering beliefs for new empowering beliefs. No longer apologising for occupying space on earth, but knowing that she deserves, like anybody else, to be here. She has decided to harness her superpower and live with an attitude of gratitude.

MESSAGE TO THE READER

Whether you are reading this at the beginning of the year, the end of the year or a random day in spring do you have some old patterns that you wish to change? Are you ready to meet your ever-changing self?

Are you ready to unveil more of who you really are? Are you ready to use your superpowers to take your life to the next level of your soul's journey?

DEDICATIONS

In memory of; Mommy May, Selina & Peggy.
Dedicated to; my Parents, my Daughter & Grand-daughters, Siblings, Nieces & Nephews.

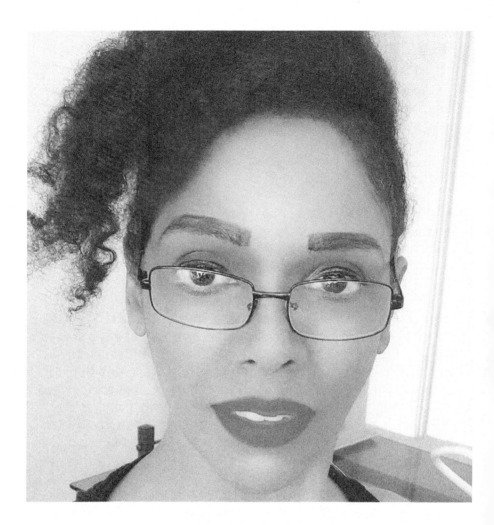

Imani Speaks

Imani Speaks

Imani Speaks is a Radio Presenter & DJ, an International Bestselling Author, an Accredited Life Coach, Certified Love Coach, a Podcaster, Health & Wellbeing Coach, Poet & Lyricist, YouTube Vlogger and Speaker.

Imani has been a Coach in many areas, since 2004 and offers intuitive support to those who need to unpack emotional pain (in a safe space), particularly in the areas of life, love and relationships and health and wellbeing.

The Imani Speaks Show and Podcast brings you interviews and conversations with talented musicians, authors, thought leaders, transformational coaches, business coaches and other community angels who are making a difference locally and globally.

Imani is a co-author in "Smashing Through The Glass Ceiling" (published in 2020) and this book too, plus she is currently working on a solo book project about the Journey of The Soul. She collaborates with singers and musicians for her poetry and lyrics and also blogs for online media organisations primarily around the areas of spirituality, personal development, love and relationships.

WEB LINKS.

Website: www.imanispeaks.com
Radio: www.conciousradio.com
Facebook: https://www.facebook.com/imanimedia
Soundcloud: https://soundcloud.com/imani-speaks
LinkedIn: https://uk.linkedin.com/in/imani-speaks-753927a6
Pinterest: https://uk.pinterest.com/imanispeaks1/boards/
Instagram: https://www.instagram.com/imanispeaks1/
YouTube: https://www.youtube.com/channel/UCRqDrqwQRXFhBg7xZm-kOwdw?view_as=public

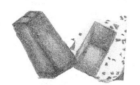

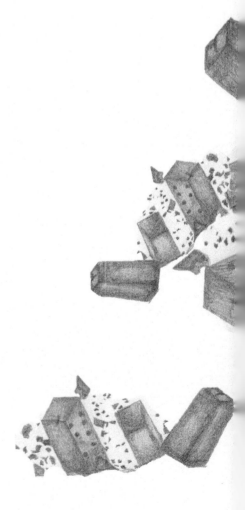

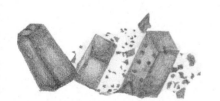

Encourage your child to always be themselves, to dream big and to talk more. Make sure they know that nothing is impossible when they believe in themselves."

~NATALIE ALLANSON

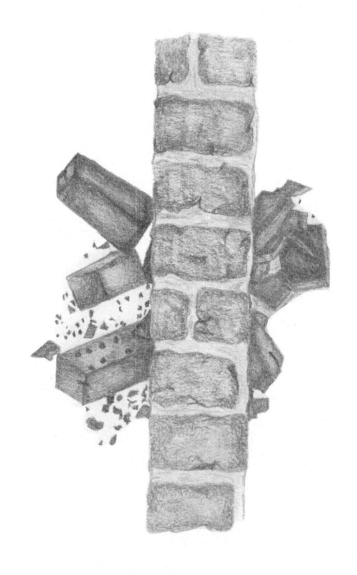

BUTTERFLIES & BULLIES

Your school years are supposed to be the happiest years of your life - carefree and full of wonder and awe at the world around you.

A llowing your curiosities to spike and your mind to expand and grow. You're a bit like a sponge in water in those early transitional days, from leaving the safety of your home and your parents care, to exploring school life and learning how to socialise with others and where you fit in the hierarchy of the school playground.

I have lots of fun and happy memories to look back on from my primary school years. My first kiss behind the bike sheds and games locker. Everyone has memories like this, can you remember what your first kiss was like? This was the kiss you'd been waiting for when you'd had a crush on a boy at school. You know the one that gave you butterflies in your tummy when he said your name. That one boy who made your legs go to jelly and your heart race all at the same time. In that one moment, nothing else mattered and time seemed to stand still. You're both that keen, you end up bumping heads or noses before you both slow down and finally lean in slowly and get it just right. Makes me cringe thinking of it now, but back then it felt magical and special and like you were the only two people in the world.

NATALIE ALLANSON

Then there was my naughty side and being sent out of class by the teacher for throwing a piece of chalk back at her when she threw it at me. I was lucky it was just the chalk. Others had the board rubber thrown at them. There was a cupboard outside the classroom that I used to stand on and pull faces through the window above the door whenever the teacher turned her back to the class, this would make everyone laugh.

> **The transition from primary school to secondary school and all the changes that came with it, both emotionally and physically, that I struggled with and I now realise that it had a massive impact on my mental health ...**

The school fairs and playing splat the rat, it was a school favourite that used to come out every year, and it always raised lots of money for the school. Who knew that a cardboard tube and a fluffy stuffed sock on a piece of string could be so much fun as you tried to whack it in the gap in the middle of the tube?

My first time on an aeroplane, if you can call it that as it was more like a shoebox with wings looking back at it now, was when I went on my first holiday away from home in year 6 to the Isle of Man. I can remember the panic I felt and the knots in my stomach, my knuckles going white as I held on tightly to the arms of the seat, the taste of the barley sugar sweet you were given to suck on to try and stop your ears from popping as you took off and climbed to new heights.

It was the transition from primary school to secondary school and all the changes that came with it, both emotionally and physically, that I struggled with and I now realise that it had a massive impact on my mental health and how I saw myself in years to come.

You see, I went from a mixed school to an all-girls secondary school, and it was a big change. I went from being happy and content to being tormented and extremely self-conscious about my body and the changes it was going through.

What should have been a beautiful time in my life transitioning from a shy quiet girl into a young woman embracing the changes within her body was marred by the cruelty of others. I no longer saw myself as a caterpillar transforming into a beautiful butterfly but more as a grub turning into a moth.

P.E. lessons were my worst nightmare, not only did you have to wear the most horrible P.E. knickers ever, (they were navy blue Bridget Jones-style pants), but you had to get changed in front of everyone and have communal showers. There were no cubicles to hide in, it was one big changing room and then a line of showers. Now back then, taking a shower was like running the gauntlet, everyone saw all your lumps and bumps and scars. You would literally run through it and get it over with as soon as possible.

If you were like me - an above-average sized girl with a well-rounded figure, you got made fun of and called cruel names. Those words stayed with me and I couldn't look myself in a mirror or take a shower without hearing them and feeling ugly and fat or "fugly" or "pigeon arse" as the bullies used to call me.

I was also an academic and I went to church, which gave the bullies something else to torment me about. The strong group of friends I had grown up with from church had all gone to different schools to me. For me, it was the name-calling and the psychological scars they left and the way those words made me feel that caused the most damage.

Words can leave more scars and can take longer to erase and heal than physical injuries sometimes. So, before you speak you should consider three things:
Is it true?
Is it necessary?
Is it kind?

and if what you're going to say doesn't tick the yes box on those three things then just don't say it.

There's an old saying that goes: "Sticks and stones may break my bones, but names will never hurt me". What a load of old codswallop that was! Names CAN hurt and I'm still dealing with the scar tissue and self-loathing they left behind – today!

Growing up I was the eldest of five, so I had no older brother or sister to look out for me. I'd always wanted a big brother growing up, someone to stand up for me and make everything ok, so I made sure I did this for my siblings though, as they grew up. There were two years between Michelle and myself and I didn't really appreciate the age gap until we were older.

> 99
> God only takes the best for his garden up there, they say...

In primary school, I was the scary big sister that would come and help her out when she had any problems with her peers. She was the annoying little sister who would borrow my stuff and who I would have to share a room with eventually as our family grew bigger. She's the sister I now miss dearly and realise just how much she meant to me growing up. You see life has a funny way of teaching us its lessons and it's only when someone or something is taken away from you, do you realise its true value and worth.

Heaven gained an angel way too soon with my sister when she gained her angel wings at 37 years of age. God only takes the best for his garden up there, they say. Well, he certainly gained a real diamond with our Shelle and I know she will be showing the rest of the angels how to have a good time up there, as well as being on my shoulder and giving me the odd kick up the backside when I need it. If you're reading this, please make sure you tell your loved ones each day how much you love and appreciate them.

Never take anyone or your life for granted as life is way too precious and it's a gift. This is the big lesson life taught me back in 2019 when we lost four people we loved dearly in the space of a few months, two of which were my Nanna and sister about 3 weeks apart.

It was like your heart was breaking over and over again and we were stuck as a family on a boat in a never-ending storm of grief. It just kept hitting us in tidal waves of gut-wrenching emotions. The fourth person we lost on the day of my sister's funeral. We questioned life, the universe and ourselves as to what we had done as a family to deserve all this pain and to be left with these gaping holes in our hearts, our lives. So, no matter what 2020 threw at me it was definitely a better year than 2019.

I can see a lot of myself and my sister in the relationship that my children, Sarah and Ryan have with each other. The squabbles and the sibling rivalry especially. However, I know they share the most amazing unbreakable bond and will always be there for each other.

Ryan is always the first person to defend his big sister and says that he will rugby tackle anyone that hurts her. Sometimes I wonder if he's older than his time and wise beyond his years. I suppose he's had to grow up quicker than most children his age through living with his medical needs.

Ryan was diagnosed with Type 1 Diabetes when he was three years old and that was the longest and loneliest night of my life. I felt truly helpless. Only one of us was allowed to stay over in the hospital when he was diagnosed, so I stayed with Ryan and Mike went home to Sarah. So many questions and "what if" scenarios went through my mind.

I blamed myself, questioned everything over and over again. Should we have picked up on it sooner? I was a support worker. "Why had I not known the signs and symptoms of Type 1 Diabetes?". Little did I know, until I got back home, that his dad was doing the same. We didn't know until the next day when the Paediatric Diabetes nurse came round the ward that there was nothing we could have done to prevent it, so for the entire night we blamed ourselves and felt guilty.

NATALIE ALLANSON

We were also told that we were lucky we caught it when we did, as had we left it any longer Ryan could have slipped into a coma in his sleep as he was in DKA (Diabetic ketoacidosis). It is caused by a lack of insulin in the body which causes a build-up of ketones in your blood turning it acidic.

Type 1 diabetes is not preventable or curable and is a lifelong condition that requires you to administer insulin via an injection or an insulin pump. In a nutshell, overnight we had become Ryan's pancreas for him, regulating his insulin intake.

Like most parents, if I could have taken it away for him and had it in his place then I would have in a heartbeat. Little did we know that 2 years later Ryan would give us another scare when he was diagnosed with Epilepsy. So, you see he's had more to deal with than most children his age. He's recently been referred back to the Epilepsy team for further investigations after he had a seizure at the table during a Sunday roast where he fell from his chair and smacked his head on the floor, just when we thought we had seen the back of the Epilepsy as he'd outgrown it. Life/ the universe never gives you more than you can handle right?!

Sarah has been our lifeline and superstar and she will never truly know how much we have appreciated her help and everything she does around the home to help us out. She has helped us with Ryan's care needs and also with babysitting too.

There was a period of time for about 3 or 4 years where we couldn't go out anywhere as a couple, due to Ryan's medical needs. It felt like we were stuck in a lockdown that only we were experiencing or in a goldfish bowl watching the world go by. It was a lot of responsibility to place on family, let alone a babysitter, and not everyone understood or could handle it.

It's not just a case of giving injections or testing his blood sugars, you have to weigh and measure out all his food and count the carbohydrate value of his food. Yes, that's right, it's the carbs we count and not the sugar content of his meals. We have to do regular night checks to make sure his blood glucose levels are in range. Ryan has no Hypo awareness whilst he's sleeping as he is such a deep sleeper. Basically, this means he doesn't wake up when his blood sugars go low, which can become life-threatening if it goes unnoticed.

We made the decision, later on, to put him on an insulin pump which gave him more freedom and also ourselves too and also meant no more injections and needles for school or us to use.
As a parent, you try and protect your children from all the bad stuff in the world and the stuff that hurt you when you were growing up. You want to wrap them up in cotton wool or put them in a giant bubble ball until they are old enough to take care of themselves. Unfortunately, you can't keep them in the goldfish bowl forever, just looking through the glass from the safety of their own little bubble.

Although with hindsight and what's been going on around us with the pandemic of 2020 that might not have been such a bad idea. You have to allow them to explore and experience the world in all its technicolour glory. That includes dealing with the bullies, a pandemic that closed the schools and colleges for over 6 months and made the entire world around go hygiene crazy. But hey, lockdown is an entirely different chapter in the story of my life and one I will save for you to read some other day.

Lunch Box Letters started out as little notes to let Ryan know how much his carbs were in his packed lunch and how much we loved him and how strong he was. As he got older, they then moved on to more positive and inspiring messages. Anything to just brighten up his school day and let him know how amazing he was, especially when he was going through tough times and he's been through a fair few of those lately.

Notes to prompt him to talk to his friends at lunchtime about their dreams and what they want to be when they grow up. To help encourage him to believe in himself and that he can do anything, especially maths when he sets his mind to it. He really doesn't like maths and thinks he can't do it, but I know he can as I have seen him do it when he gives it a go and tries his best.
Some people may think I am making him soft by putting notes in his lunch box and think it's daft, but when he comes home with a

big smile on his face and says thank you for his lunch and the note I left him, I know it's worthwhile and has been a good day for him. Ryan is even sharing the letters with his friends and they ask him can they read them. I know there will come a point in his life when he starts secondary school, that he no longer wants them in his lunch box and I will start to send them as text messages or emails instead or just ring his mobile on his way to school like I do with Sarah when she is on her way to college.

Writing a lunchbox letter is just one way we can all encourage our children to always be themselves and to dream big. To talk more and know that nothing is impossible when you believe in yourself. It's a way of letting them know that you believe in them and love them no matter what, that all you ask is they do their best. That it's ok to be different, everyone has their own unique qualities and flaws. It's what makes us so flawsome and amazing. Let's face it the world would be a very boring place if we were all the same shade of beige.

It's ok if your son wants to wear pink and grow their hair and likewise, if your daughter wants to play with action men and climb trees. Boys can do ballet just as much as girls can play football. Teach your children to see the individual and not the stereotype or label, to lead with kindness and love in everything they do and to smile more and laugh lots.

DEDICATION

I have decided to dedicate this chapter firstly to anyone that has ever been made to feel worthless or told they won't amount to anything or that they don't belong.

To anyone that has been bullied or is being bullied. Don't be afraid of asking for help or letting your light shine. You are amazing and you will get through this. Learn from your experiences and keep moving forward, only look back to see how much you have grown.

Secondly, I dedicate this to my sister who I wrote about in my chapter. She was and still is one of the strongest women and true warrior queens I have ever known. She continues to be the angel on my shoulder kicking my ass every day and that voice that comes from nowhere and encourages me to stand up for myself and to keep sharing my story and lifting others up along the way. You were always there for your family despite fighting demons of your own. You never gave up. You were our rock, and we all miss you dearly.

Michelle Louise Allanson
1981 - 2019

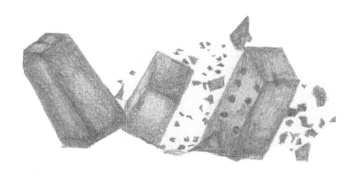

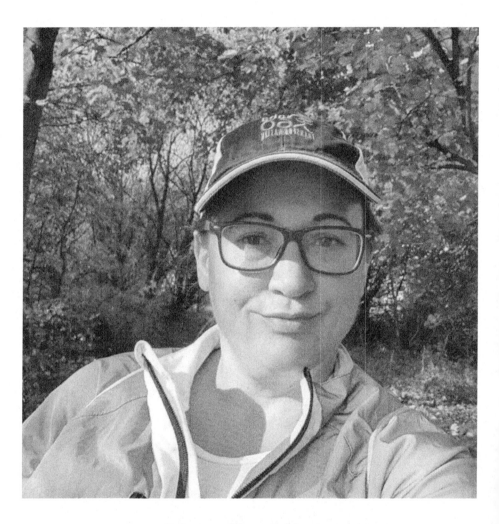

Natalie Allanson

Natalie Allanson

Natalie was recently listed as the UK's Top 100 women in cycling. She is also a Network Marketer, Motivator and Volunteer.
She is a Mum of 3 and one of her children has Type 1 Diabetes, so Natalie is an advocate for that too.
She wants to change the world one smile at a time, and she is passionate about working with special needs families. Natalie is a qualified Health and Social Care Worker and Mental Health Worker.
Natalie has also recently launched her podcast and her blog.

Social Media Links:
Facebook - https://www.facebook.com/Natalie.Allanson
Blog - https://lupusmum.blogspot.com
Podcast - https://anchor.fm/natalie-allanson

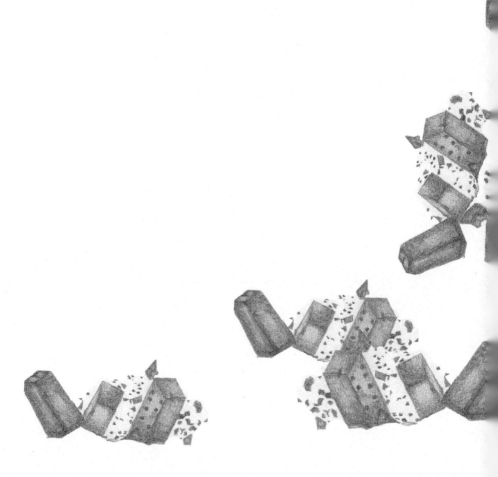

No matter what you're
going through or to whom
took you through it,
if you're standing
on faith – your foundation
is solid"

~CHEVALA HARDY

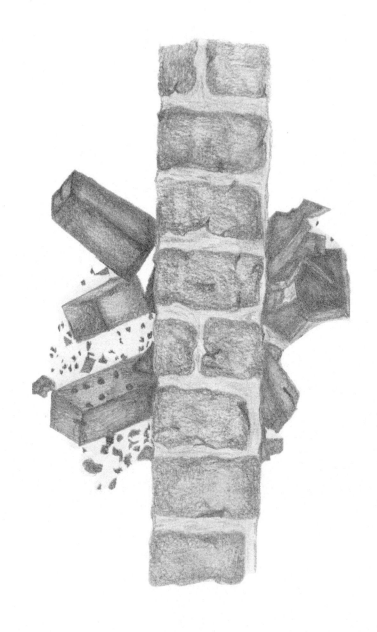

The Secret Keeper

Gazing out the window, listening to the rain drops on my metal roof and thinking about all the conversations I've had with my mom, all I hear in my head are the times she said to me, "you were a mistake", "yes I love your sister more than you", "you'll never be anything".

Can you just imagine, as a child, this is the only memory you have and some teen years and the rest are that of a ghost?

Remembering the no support in school activities and the bouncing from house to house. I remember my mother told me that my real dad was an alcoholic and he came in and made her have sex one night from what she tells me, so that's basically rape. My mom had only just had my sister about 8 months when she got pregnant with me.

Putting this all together now can explain why she hates me.
My mother didn't really raise me. I spent a lot of time at different places growing up. I don't really remember my childhood with my mother at all and I don't know if my life has been suppressed from

all of the bad memories or if is it a blockage in my mind.
I have never felt the love that I should feel from a parent even to this day.

This takes me to my very first memory I have when I was a child. I was about 5 years old and I was living with my Uncle. I loved being there because my cousin used to play this game with me and my prize was candy.

He taught me how to become The Secret Keeper!

He would take me in this room by the kitchen and make me take a nap and the things he did to me when I got older I found out weren't right but he had taught me how to become a great secret keeper at age 5.

It didn't stop there!

As i got older i found that in the family that was a normal thing among the guys. They liked to sit me on their laps and touch on me just for their own gratification and tell me to keep it a secret.

I kinda feel they all knew I was abandoned by my mom and used me as a target.

I guess you can say that my story is all over the place and it is because at that time my life was all over the place and the memories that I have I try not to have. Telling a story of this kind is hard but necessary when your goal is to help someone that has experienced the same.

Have you ever just tried to find a happy childhood moment and couldn't?

So, I finally found a place to call home with my Grandparents. I was as happy as i could ever imagine.

My Grandparents treated me just like I was their own child. I received the love from them that I had been missing for almost 12 years of my life. I had great meals and I went to lots of different family functions. Even though I love my mother and I would never allow anyone to disrespect her.

I met a guy at a skating rink one night. He was a very nice gentleman to me and very kind. He was much older than me and I used to see him around and we used to talk a lot and he listened to me and he became my best friend.

I told this guy about how my mom neglected me and how I was moved from house to house and all the gruesome details of my life. He told me he would be there for me, how he would never hurt me, and he always hugged me, so he started to come visit me at school.

I thought that was very cool. I finally had a friend to love. He never touched me to make me uncomfortable and I always felt safe and that's what I loved about him. He did get up the nerve to kiss me one time and I was okay with that because I liked him a lot.

I was so happy with my life and I was doing well in school. My grandmother put me into dance class and then my mom made me come home...

That was the worst thing that could ever happen to me.

> "All of the madness started all over again ... all of the mental abuse, all of the emotional abuse, everything!!!

All of the madness started all over again - all of the mental abuse, all of the emotional abuse, everything!!! It was like my mom just wanted me to live in sadness all of my life and I didn't understand why she wanted me to be unhappy.

My mom's husband had to bring his 2 boys to live with us for some reason. Present time makes me wonder if one of the boys touched their sisters in an inappropriate manner.

CHEVALA HARDY

They saw how I was being mistreated all this time by my mother. They were aware that I wasn't loved and also that I was being mentally abused and very mistreated.

What I know now, that I didn't understand then as I was only 13 years old, was that my daddy had raped her and that's why she didn't like me. My grandmother was so heartbroken, and she felt like she had lost her child and I felt like I had lost my mother because we were so close. I was lost all over again.

> "
> My grandmother was so heartbroken, and she felt like she had lost her child and I felt like I had lost my mother...

My Brother?

I felt like Cinderella as I used to be the one to be made to clean up all the time and everything. I hated being at home. I just wanted to be back with my grandmother. But, I believe, that's why my mom made me come back home because I was happy there and she did not like me being happy and doing good.

My parents were gamblers and they were gone from the home all the time. My mom would leave on a Friday and I would not see her until she got home from work on Monday sometimes.

It was the holidays, no one was home at the time but us kids and this life changing secret happened to me.....

Early Christmas morning, I was awakend to my oldest brother having sex with me. OH My Goodness

I didn't understand this. Besides being scared all i could think of was what did i do to deserve this.

"Every young lady that thinks of her first love encounter never imagines this"

Afterwards, I was crying from fear and pain. Can you imagine saving yourself for the person you think you love and until you feel you're ready and then that dream gets taken away and by a sibling? I sat on the bed which was the top bunk feeling nasty and confused. After all, who could I tell anyways?

After I stopped beating myself up I got down to go get in the shower. Oh the pain I felt from standing was horrible. I got in the shower and turned it on as hot as I could stand it and the crying started all over again.

I could not believe that this had just happened to me!

I wanted my mom so bad but I knew she would not even care and find a way to blame me for what happened and I was just in my bed asleep. So this would just be another one of my secrets that nobody had to know about so i thought.

Over the years many questions have run through my head. Was it rape? Was it molestation? Was it consensual because I didn't speak out or stop him? Was it rape and molestation? At that time i didnt even know those words' meanings. I mean I was 13 years old and fast asleep and woke with him forcing himself onto me. He was my brother, and he did what he did, but would anyone believe me? What could I do? What could they do?

I was in love with my friend who I saw at my grandmothers, the person who listened to me, the one who we spoke for hours together. He was who I wanted to be with - my first time. So, keeping the secret of what just happened to me I called my friend and told him I was ready to be with him so later that day he picked me up and he took me to his place where we went to his room and he put me gently on the bed and started to kiss me. He made me relax and as I was only 13 years old, I just wanted someone to love me. That's all I wanted as I didn't get love from my mom. I thought this time would be the perfect love story.

Typical thinking from an emotional broken 13 year old! I honestly believe at this point I was just a broken, hurt, and confused little girl with lots of secrets.

To be perfectly honest after it was over, I forgot all about it and he forgot about me. I don't remember hearing from him or seeing him that much after this happened and that broke my heart all over again.

Was this another setup for me? Was this really a prepping for him to get what he wanted from me? Was this another one of his schemes and he just played me all alone just because I was a vulnerable young girl from a broken home? What was this really?

Talking about a double whammy!

So, I made myself just forget all about him because I had got so used to being let down by everyone; it was just my way of life. I just decided to keep it all a secret and move on.

I honestly believe God made me with a built in memory blocker for my protection!

My older brother started to be nice and I just figured that was just because he didn't want me to tell anyone about what he had done to me but I didn't care - it was all over and done with and I really didn't even think about that because it really didn't matter to me anyway.

Want to know something crazy? That little that didn't get any love started to like that niceness because that was the only niceness she was getting even though it was fake.

What a life for a kid!
I didn't think about guys anymore. I just wanted to live my life, go to school, run track and just be a better me, but I started to feel sick. I didn't know what was going on. I just wanted to lay around and I was tired all the time. I was falling asleep in school. I just didn't feel good.

I was very small and very petite and very short. I didn't know much because my mom didn't tell me a whole lot and I didn't really have a lot of friends, but I just knew something was wrong. So, I decided to go to the health department as I didn't really have a reason to be on birth control because I wasn't doing anything but my whole life changed in that moment that I was told I was pregnant! 13 years old and pregnant - how was going to tell my mom? How was I going to be able to keep this ultimate secret!

I honestly did not know about pregnancy. I was confused. I felt alone and scared. I just did not know what to do. So, the first thing that I did was to write my older brother a letter about what he had done to me that morning. He never responded and the next thing I know my daddy moved my brothers to their grandparents.

It does make me wonder if he told his dad and showed him the letter, so dad wanted him to leave the house and then join the military to straighten him out because that's exactly what he did. I also contacted my long-lost love to let him know that at 14 years of age I was pregnant.

With two possible fathers and a mother that hated me now more than ever for being pregnant at a young age what chance did I have? I still kept a secret from my mom and I felt like my mom or my stepdad kept a secret from me - that they knew that my brother did what he did to me and they didn't do anything about it but just move him out of the house. And, I have thought that if this was the original behaviour of why they moved in with us from California in the first place, then she, as my mom should have made it clear that they weren't allowed near the girls and kept them away from me and my sisters completely.

> " I honestly believe God made me with a built in memory blocker for my protection!

CHEVALA HARDY

Later, I found out that he had also done this to my other sister too, but it was too late. He had already done the damage to me - physically, mentally, and emotionally.

As a child you are unaware of things like this until you grow up and see why you act and respond the way you do.

Often at times in our life, we get caught up in physical attraction, emotional attachment, and the desires to be loved that we don't see the mental disaster that we cause to ourselves but what do we know at the age of 13? I was in love with a guy older than me that I had slept with after my brother did what he did to me. I wasn't thinking straight but I was only a child.

Thave accepted the fact that none of this was my fault. We often look for love in the wrong places when we're young. I thank God that my grandmother brought me up in the church and that God has given me a forgiving heart, a loving heart and direction. I don't hold anything against these guys. I always let God fight my battles because vengeance is the Lord's. I love everyone and I wish everyone well.

Yes, I was hurt but I worked through all of the pain. It took some time but with God all things are possible.

I have for years helped others and decided to pursue a career as a professional life coach. In doing this I aim to help others get through similar and same situations just as I have. together we can win.

This is my story of how I was trained from age 5 and up to be The Secret Keeper has made me the strong woman I am today. I pray that if anyone has gone through any such trauma that I've experienced that they will reach out and we can work through this together.

You Are Not Alone - God is with all of us. I love you and I pray God's blessings upon you always.

The Secret Keeper

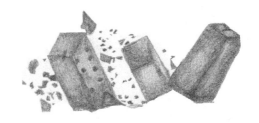

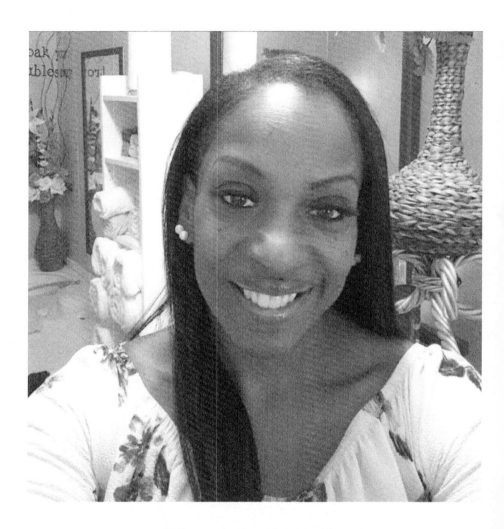

Chevala Hardy

Chevala Hardy

Forced to become a mother at age 14, another at 15, 17 and 19 she still finished school and managed to go to college and land a few jobs and then was fired and that inspired her to want to tell her life story in writing.

She has recently finished her course in NLP and Hypnosis to jumpstart her Life Coaching Business. She is a licensed insurance agent and she also owns her own transportation business. Her passion is to help others.

Chevala hopes in telling her story and being vulnerable, it will encourage the readers to reach out and speak up if they have been through the same experience. Her main message is that "no matter how hard life seems, if you stand firm on your faith you will always win".

She lives in Georgia, USA.

Website & SM Links:

Facebook https://www.facebook.com/chevala.hardy

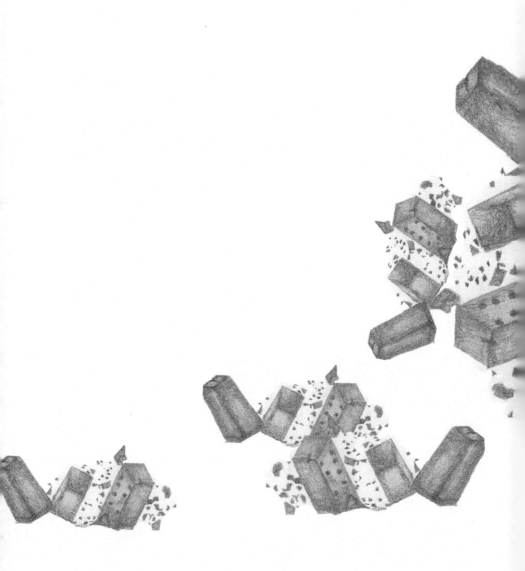

Lying there helpless in
a hospital bed,
unable to move, see,
eat or care for myself.
Unbearable pain
searing through my
head.
Will I have tomorrow?"

~MICHELLE ROCHE

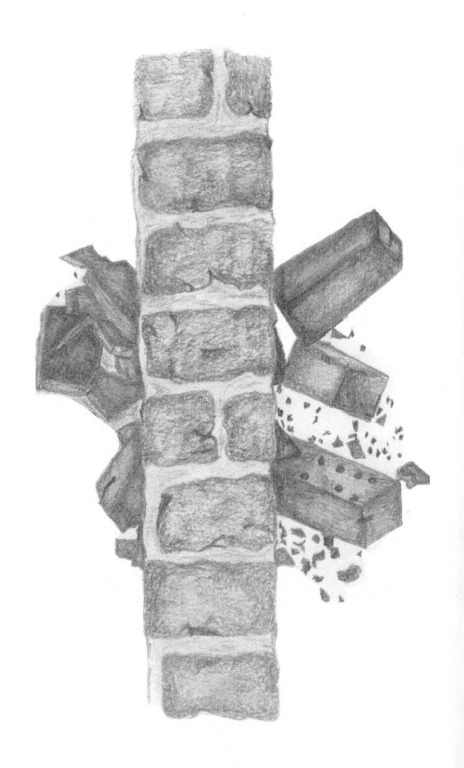

The Pyramid Inside My Brain

"BIG MISTAKE - the pain hit me like a lightning bolt all over again".

Throughout my life I have suffered with horrendous migraine headaches. The older I got the worse they would be and often last two to three days at a time. They always came on very suddenly, my stomach would turn, and my mouth would water and then the almighty pain in my head would erupt.

I would often use Reiki on myself to relieve the symptoms of my persistent migraines. It did provide me with some relief, but I was still suffering a couple of migraines a month, each one lasting a couple days at a time. I lost a lot of my life to migraine headaches. I'd been told from childhood that the headaches I suffered were migraine headaches and, as my Mum was also a sufferer, I never questioned it.

Around 2008 my migraines became more frequent but less severe. It was in this year that, together with my parents, a holiday to Florida was planned. Both of my daughters had a fabulous time, so much so, that we did it again the following year. On both occasions I had a persistent headache. I put it down to the heat and humidity. It wasn't like my typical migraine but more of a dull ache that just wouldn't go away.

In 2011, I began experiencing more severe migraines. The pain was so unbearable, and my head would feel sore and bruised for days afterward. They were always on the left side of my head and no amount of pain relief helped in any way.

Sunday 4th November 2012 is a day that I will never forget!

I'd recently re-connected with a friend from my clubbing days. We found each other on Facebook and had arranged a catch up. On the short drive back home, I experienced the usual onset of a migraine. My mouth began to water, and I knew I needed to be sick. "Not in my car, please don't let me be sick in my car", I repeatedly said to myself.

> "Not in my car, please don't let me be sick in my car", I repeatedly said to myself...

Then the headache came - like a bolt of lightning in my head. I was just five minutes from home. "I can do this", I said to myself, and I did. Once through the front door I moved as fast as I could to the kitchen sink. Crawling up the stairs I made my way to bed. My daughters were with their Dad, so it was just me and my furry, four legged, loyal companions.

The following morning, I was pretty much in the same state, which was nothing new for me. It was now Bonfire night and I remember all too well the sounds of the fireworks going off outside. I shuddered with each loud bang, lying in my bed afraid to make any movements, as moving triggered the urge to wretch, which in turn caused more pain. I stayed like this for the following three days.

It was now Wednesday, and I felt a slight improvement. So, I took the opportunity to have a shower.
BIG MISTAKE - the pain hit me like a lightning bolt all over again.

The vomiting returned and I was back to square one. My partner at the time had come to stay, he tried to look after me but to be fair there wasn't much he could do. At least he could take care of my dogs. My symptoms had begun to change, and I was experiencing symptoms not typical of my migraines. My vision was blurry, and everything hurt - even my fingers and toes.

Friday morning came and I was feeling very poorly. My partner popped his head into the bedroom to say he was going to work. He left and I was alone with my dogs, but I knew I needed to get some help, so on my hands and knees I crawled from my bed. Unable to stand, my balance was gone but I had to find my phone. Crawling across the landing I found my phone. I managed to ring my parents. My mum answered and knew instantly I was unwell. Luckily, we lived close to each other and they were with me in no time. My Dad took one look at me and said, "We need to take you to hospital".

The journey was horrendous, I've never felt so poorly. The movement of the car was agonising, and the blurry vision didn't help the constant urge to vomit. Finally, we arrived in A&E and I was wheeled into a cubicle.

I don't remember everything, but I remember being given some medication. It was just after 8am and I remained in hospital until they discharged me at around 9pm. Having been seen by three consultants I was given the diagnosis of severe migraine. In fact, the words they used were "It's nothing more than a severe migraine" and so my parents reluctantly wheeled me out through the hospital waiting room. My Dad drove his car as near to the door as he could, and they took me back home with them.

Here I was back in my old bedroom, my parents worried out of their minds, trying their best to care for me. The pain I was in was like nothing I'd ever experienced in my life before. I'd gone through two labours with no more than gas & air and I'd take that again over this pain any day. Throughout it all I felt so sorry for my family, especially my parents. As poorly as I was, I could see the anguish in their faces every time they came in the room to check on me. It wasn't until the following Wednesday and two further visits to A&E that I finally had a CT scan.

MICHELLE ROCHE

My Mum and my sister had been to see my GP and literally begged him to refer me for a scan. He instructed them to ring 999 for an ambulance, which they did. After an hour or so in A&E, I was taken onto the admissions ward where I spent the night. By this time my vision was double, and I was very unsteady on my feet. I recall my sister taking me to the bathroom and having to literally sit me down on the toilet.

At some time during the night, I was examined by a Junior Doctor who actually listened to what I was saying. By this time, I was seeing all kinds of amazing things, from a fox cub running around my bed to a little boy in a box playing with a train set. There were gold murals dancing on the walls and ceiling and everything looked so bright. I could see a man in the bed next to me who was made of paper. I knew that no one else could see what I was seeing but everything was so clear and real to me. My Mum and Sister stayed with me until the early hours of the morning.

The consultant came to do his morning round and told me I was due to have a CT scan at midday. He then said I'd be able to "get off home afterwards!'. The feeling of complete helplessness is very difficult to put into words, my life was literally in the hands of others. I knew there was something very seriously wrong within me and those that know me best knew it too.

My Mum and sister were back by my bedside and there they stayed. A porter came with a wheelchair to take me for my scan. My sister came with me and as I was being wheeled back to the ward, I was telling her about the dancing gold bears I was seeing, I'm not sure what the porter thought! Both my parents and my sister were sat by my bedside when, yet another consultant, came to discuss the scan results.

"Some abnormality", "a bleed on the brain". These were the words I heard as I looked at the faces of my loved ones. For me there was a sense of relief. I knew how poorly I was, and I no longer had to convince the Doctors.
Eventually I was transferred by ambulance to Salford Royal Foundation Trust where I had a further CT scan followed by an angiogram. The result was that I'd had a Subarachnoid brain haemorrhage. The angiogram showed the healing process had begun, and

proved the haemorrhage happened around 7 to 10 days previously. The usual procedure is to have coils fitted inside the aneurysm. An aneurysm is normally shaped like a berry but mine was shaped more like a pyramid. (In layman's terms they needed some kind of scaffolding to bridge the gap in the artery).

I was told that the only thing stopping further bleeding was a scab that had formed along the ruptured artery wall. The most upsetting moment was about to unfold, seeing my Dad's face crumple as he said to the nurse "so the only thing stopping the bleeding is a scab"?

Heart-breaking……. just heart-breaking.

I wanted to sit up and put my arms around him and tell him that I was going to be fine, but I couldn't. Lying there helpless, unable to move, but feeling so many emotions and the realisation that they could be faced the very real possibility of losing me.

When you're faced with the very real possibility of your existence coming to an end you truly understand the meaning of life. I spent weeks lying in a hospital bed with nothing to do but think and listen. I listened to what was going on around me. I heard others being told that there was nothing more could be done for them. One lady in particular stays with me to this day. I heard her break down, the sound of the heart wrenching sobs long after the doctors had left her bedside. She walked past my bed and stopped. Our eyes locked, and she said "Michelle, there's nothing they can do for me". What could I say? Nothing, I had no words, my eyes filled, and the tears spilled out and rolled down my cheeks.

> "Lying there helpless, unable to move, but feeling so many emotions and the realisation that they could be faced the very real possibility of losing me...

MICHELLE ROCHE

Lying there, thoughts turned to my family, my loved ones, my daughters, my parents and as I was unable to see properly and unable to eat, it made me feel sad. I couldn't even have any flowers to cheer me up, as I was on a surgical ward. My wonderful work colleagues did club together to buy me a box of chocolates, books and a beautiful bouquet of flowers. Typical isn't it, oh the irony, anyway nothing went to waste. My daughters enjoyed the chocolates, and the flowers and books went home with my family.

Meanwhile the team looking after me were busy sending my scan pictures around the world. They didn't know what to do for me and it was the French who came up with a solution. They had developed a carbon stent two years previously. It was decided that this would be purchased and brought over by a surgeon who would assist in my operation. What a relief!

> I had good days and bad days. The pain went from horrendous to bearable. Being on morphine caused a whole lot of other problems. I won't go into detail...

December 6th was the day of my op and until then I just had to sit tight and wait. I had good days and bad days. The pain went from horrendous to bearable. Being on morphine caused a whole lot of other problems. I won't go into detail, but I can assure you I will never ever have another enema as long as I live. It was one of the worst experiences of my life.

The evening of the operation arrived. My daughters were arguing over who was going to sit on the comfy chair. One of the surgical team arrived to discuss the procedure, explaining everything in detail to me and my family. All I could do was look at their faces and feel their anguish.

I only asked one question, "how long will it take?"
The answer, "It will take as long as it takes, we will not be rushing that's for sure!"

It was explained that the drugs I'd been given over the last couple of days, to thin my blood, meant they wouldn't be able to stop any bleeding. The morning came and the vascular surgeon came to introduce himself and went through the whole procedure. After he left, I rang my parents. My Dad answered the phone, and I couldn't speak. He knew it was me and kept saying my name I gulped several times - the emotion hit me hard!! It could be the last time I will ever speak to my parents. Then the team arrived with the trolley to transfer me to theatre and so off I went.

As I opened my eyes, I noticed the clock on the wall - 1.15 pm and then I was aware of a strange sensation in my legs. A nurse was talking to me, "I've just rang your parents" she said. I was in the recovery room and all had gone according to plan.

My throat was so dry, and I was worried about the sensation in my legs. I asked the nurse if I could have some water and what was wrong with my legs? The sensation I was feeling was caused by an Intermittent pneumatic compression (IPC) device to prevent blood clots forming in the deep veins of the legs.

The relief was immense as I thought they'd made some kind of mistake and chopped my legs off instead. Joking aside, the team had performed a remarkable job. I was moved onto the high dependency unit where I remained for two days. Amazing to think that a tiny stent was inserted into my right femoral artery and ended up in the carotid artery on the left side of my brain, amazing!!

The day after the surgery I was experiencing a lot of pain as the operation had caused my vessels to go into spasm causing headaches and vomiting. Thankfully this only lasted a day, and on the Saturday, two days after surgery, I was back on the ward.

Hearing my daughters say they're going to have to spend Christmas Day in hospital gave me the strength I needed. No way was that happening! I would be home way before Christmas and so, with that positive mindset and determination, I made a pretty miraculous recovery. On Monday the 10th of December I was on my way home, only four days after my surgery.

The road to recovery carried on long after I was discharged from the hospital. Tired had a whole new meaning to me. It was a tired I'd never experienced before. Looking back, I know I did too much too soon. I remember shopping in the supermarket and the strange sensation it gave me. Like my brain just couldn't process all the information thrown at it.

I created a filing cabinet in my head to help me to remember words I'd forgotten. I would file a word away, so I'd remember where it was if I forgot it again. I know how lucky I am to have survived and to have no permanent brain damage. I was angry at the way I was treated in A&E and the patronising tone of the medical staff. I was angry that my parents had to go through the trauma of looking after me when I was so very poorly.

The thing that played on my mind the most was the thought of someone else going through the same thing. For this reason, I decided to make an official complaint to the hospital. Many people have asked why I didn't sue them. Maybe if I had been left with permanent damage I would have had to. All I wanted was for them to learn from the mistakes they made and for no one else to have to suffer the way I did.

We know our bodies better than anyone else and if I had been given a CT scan when I first presented in A&E I would not have suffered in pain for as long as I did. Oh, and as for the migraines, I no longer suffer from them. Again, what amazing relief!

During my recovery I found I was writing more. Poetry began to flow, and I'd started to draw again. My creativity continued to grow, and I began painting and trying different mediums. Painting eyes became a theme, and this has continued to be the case. This can be seen in much of the artwork inspired by partner's song writing.

Our joint creativity is continuing to grow. I am thankful every day for all I have, to my family for taking such good care of me and fighting my corner when I was unable to. I think this is a good place to end this chapter of my story.

DEDICATION.
I dedicate this chapter to my parents Kath and Mike for always taking such great care of me.
To my daughters Ella and Georgia for making me laugh through the pain. To my sister Karen for the personal care and pampering and to everyone else who showed me love and support.
I'm so grateful to you all and I love you all dearly.

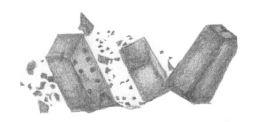

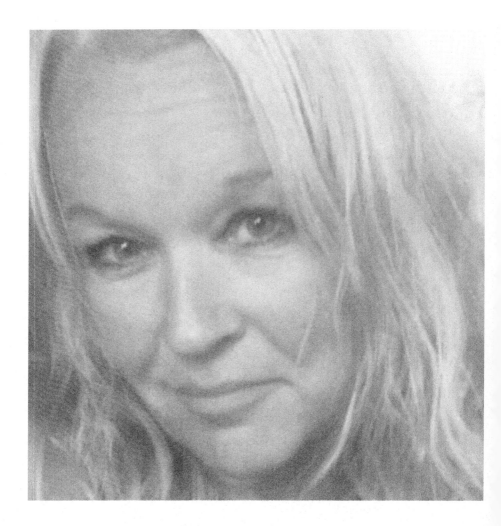

Michelle Roche

Michelle Roche

Michelle has worked in the caring profession for over 25yrs. Many of those were with the NHS, caring for new mothers and their babies. It was during her time working for the NHS that she became increasingly interested in Holistic Therapies. Through her work in Maternity Services she was able to study Auricular Acupuncture.

From there, Michelle went on to study Reiki and has been a Reiki Practitioner since 2007. In 2008, she achieved a Diploma in Indian Head Massage and a year later a Diploma in Thai Foot Massage. She also spent two years studying Homeopathy at the North West College of Homeopathy. In 2012, Michelle had a life-changing experience. Having been a migraine sufferer since childhood, severe headaches were part of normal life for her.

After waking up one morning, with what she thought was another severe migraine, Michelle took her usual action. This time though things would be very different. After several visits to A&E, a CT scan twelve days later revealed the truth. Michelle had suffered a Subarachnoid Brain Haemorrhage caused by a ruptured aneurysm.

After making a full recovery Michelle rediscovered her love of creativity. Painting and drawing was something she loved to do in her youth. As with many of us, work and family life take up much of our time, leaving less time for our true passions.

Michelle believes that having a near death experience makes you look at life slightly differently. Since 2013 she has been working towards combining her passion for creativity with earning an income and helping as many people as she can along the way.

LINKS.
www.facebook.com/michelle.roche.5602
www.facebook.com/Chelles-Crafts-2056856191223916

EMAIL
MRcreations300@gmail.com

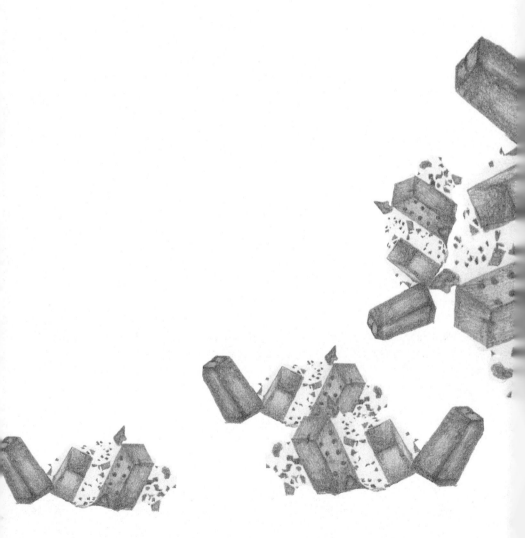

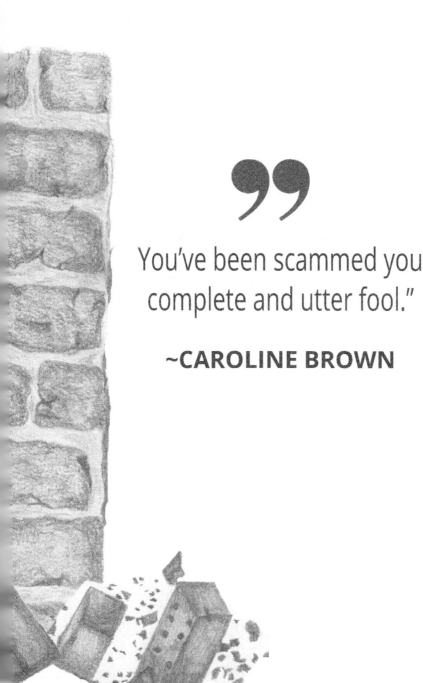

99

You've been scammed you complete and utter fool."

~CAROLINE BROWN

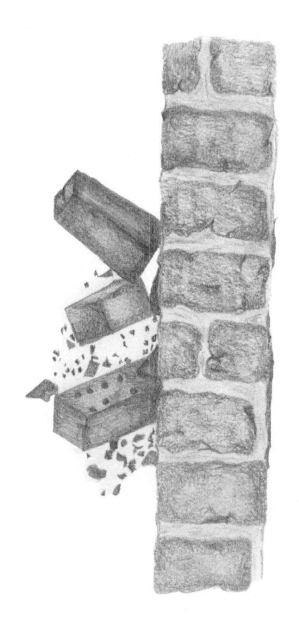

Making it out of the pit of despair...

"You've been scammed you complete and utter fool"

A s those words were screaming at me from inside my own head, from within my own gut, and ripping at my entire soul sank in, I truly, at that point, loathed and despised myself so much that I felt I was drowning in my own agony.

The hatred and anger that I felt towards myself was all consuming. The realisation that I had been made a fool of, had had my strings well and truly pulled like a lifeless, inanimate, and farcical puppet, and was probably being laughed at for how easy I had been to manipulate made me want to rip my own heart out.

You see, I had become desperate. Not desperate at first, but the eager anticipation of the better life I would have for myself and my children if I joined this company, that company, this affiliate programme, that affiliate programme, this person's or that person's business, after about 5 years gave way to the grim realisation that not only was I no better off, certainly wasn't my own boss, financially or time free like all these people had promised was mine for the taking, rather I was significantly out of pocket, and pretty much running out of hope!

CAROLINE BROWN

My story, if you will, began in Brighton in 1963 when I was born, not that I remember much about that! I grew up with my sister, with our mum and dad. I loved where I lived, loved being by the sea, and have many happy memories of growing up. We used to have holidays to Hungary and Romania usually every couple of years or so which were incredible. My mum was from Hungary, and had relatives in Budapest, and in The Carpathian Mountains and other remote spots in Romania. That is where my love affair with travelling abroad was born.

> **My early 20s, travelling abroad was really all I wanted to do...**

My memories of long, warm, fun days at the beaches in Brighton & Hove as children are so precious and very happily a part of who I am, but I was so romanced by the whole travelling to distant lands experiences (though it was Europe, it did seem a distant land to me as a child). Although I didn't actually realise it at the time, it made such an impact on me, when I got into my early 20s, travelling abroad was really all I wanted to do.

I left Brighton at the age of 20, to pursue a career in Nursing up in Surrey. A very nice old market town, on the River Thames. Many happy years - the best years of my life workwise were spent in Nursing in various locations, always in this country. As we all know, things happen in life which we don't necessarily expect or plan.

My precious children came along, and they are truly the love of my life, all of them. The history there is not necessary to go into, but I ended up pretty much a single mum, with the exception of my youngest child's dad who did his best to support us. We weren't compatible to live together, and his jobs were never really stable. But he did try.

I was just over 40 when I decided that my youngest child was settled well in school, and it was time I went back to work. I was lucky enough to get a job in retail, part time at first. I decided against going back to nursing for several reasons. Not least of which was the 8 months Back to Nursing course I would have to complete but also pay a lot to do! I was happy enough in my new job at first, grateful to be back in the workplace, grateful to be "of use" as I felt to society!

But this is where the story changes. It didn't take long before I started to start feeling very uncomfortable in my job. I had worked hard to climb up the ladder, so to speak. I moved departments after 3 months and realised it would be pretty straightforward to become one under the Manager. So, I went about becoming his right hand, quietly, but purposefully. Usually when I put my mind to something, I get it done. So, it was - I did. For a few years it was quite fulfilling really, no comparison to the fulfilment I always got from my years of Nursing in the hospital, but I made some changes, implemented ideas I knew would make the Department more productive, and threw myself into the job.

Old Father Time, who waits for no man or woman started to move faster and faster, and before I knew it, I was 50! Not a problem, I told myself, in fact I congratulated myself for getting this far all things considered! But I was restless. I was becoming increasingly more frustrated and disillusioned with my job. So, I started my journey of seeking a way out of the desperation that I felt being locked into. The ever increasingly unattractive, stifling, unfulfilling and financially lack filled future I was facing if I carried on the same dismal path.

I'd followed a few people online - leaders in their field of online businesses. The picture portrayed was that of halcyon days, and ultimate freedom. Yes, they all said you have to work hard to begin with, but put in the work, and the rewards will come. Oh, and of course, "you don't need to spend a lot of money".

Please let me be crystal clear here - there are genuine people out there with their own online businesses, who are successful through their own merit, hard graft, determination and powerful mindsets. I think I was just looking at the wrong people, in the wrong places. Not that these people I was being influenced by were not successful, it's just that I was too easily seduced by all the promises that it didn't occur to me to do any research - no, I jumped in with my eyes closed, wallet open, hope in heart, but totally gullible!

October 2018
After yet another failed attempt at making an online 'opportunity' work out positively for me, and having poured yet more money down the drain, the anger and frustration were so big and corrupting inside of me that I lost all sense of perspective. I lost all sense of logic, all sense full stop! I cannot describe the feelings of inadequacy and incompetence that resulted in me doing the stupidest thing ever.

Flicking through social media as one does, I came across a post which detailed how money could be made and made fast in the crypto currency space. It featured an interview with a couple on a daytime news programme who had seen their investment grow ridiculously during the time of their programme being on air - about 2 hours. They had only invested about £200 and ended up with a few thousand £ by the end of their broadcast.

Gullible as I was, I thought that it was a legitimate interview. Desperate as I was, I clicked on the link that supposedly would take me to the place online where I could do the same as what I had seen happen on the post I had just looked at. I did hesitate, but not for long. Not once did I listen to my gut instinct. Right then, I was beyond all rationality, and beyond all capacity to listen to it. I count at least two red flags at this point which I should have seen!

I was taken to a completely different online site altogether to the one I had been expecting. Slightly confused, but nonetheless completely determined, not to mention rather deranged I can safely say, I continued. Third red flag should have been when I realised that the minimum investment was not £200 like they had led me to believe on the post, but in fact £1000. Alright, I thought to myself, I'm here now, might as well get on with it! I deposited the £1000, after filling in my details - name, phone number, email - the usual. Within about two minutes, I received a phone call.

The call was from a man with an Eastern European accent. He was very friendly, very engaging, and very convincing. His "honied" words worked their magic. He told me his name, where he was originally from, and that he was one of the senior account managers of the company whose website I was on. He explained how the system worked - my deposit would be put to work on trading Bitcoin against the USD and against other crypto currencies. Fourth red flag... he said that £1000 was okay, but I would make more, faster, if I was to up my deposit to £3000 in total. Like a fool I did as he suggested. Had I been I overtaken by complete madness, or greed, or both? Complete madness yes, greed? It certainly sounds like it doesn't it! Yes, I wanted money, and yes, I wanted it fast. I wanted money so I could do what I'd been trying to do for a few years and leave my mind-numbing job. I wanted it so I could be my own boss, and live life on my terms. I wanted it so I could take my kids on holidays, my grandkids on holidays. I wanted it so I could travel to far distant lands. I wanted it to help others, to give to people that had nothing - clean water, lifesaving medicines, education, freedom from tyranny... I wanted it to be free so I could do all these things.

> **Gullible as I was, I thought that it was a legitimate interview...**

I logged in to my desktop, and I shared my screen with him. I know, a total stranger right!! He showed me where to place the initial trade, and then told me to log out, and he would take care of the trade from thereon in. As I find all things crypto confusing, it was somewhat comforting that all the technical stuff was going to be taken off my hands and 'managed' by the expert. My own trading account manager!!

He promised to call me in a day or two with an update of how the trade went, and how much "we" had made. Fifth red flag? True to his promise, he called. He said we had made over $6000 (my investment was in GBP, but for purposes of trading, the currency was USD). I was absolutely delighted, of course!! I asked for my share to be deposited back to my bank account. He wasn't having any of that. I'm going to stop counting red flags at this point. Suffice it to say that yes it was another one! I asked him why not, and he just said that we would make so much money if I let him use the profits on another trade. I told him I wasn't happy, and I would rather have some of the profits in my bank account, but he used psychological manipulation on me, and so I caved. Another trip to the desktop and the trade was placed.

Once again, he promised to call me in a few days. I had a number for him and an email address for him, so I wasn't too worried that he was going to run off with my money. I started getting a bit worried when he didn't call, so I eventually tried to call him. I got through to a lady who called herself his PA. She told me that she would get him to call me. Eventually he did, but he sounded irritated on the phone. Another red flag!! I asked him why he hadn't called, and he just said he had been busy, and that there was nothing to report on the trade. He said it hadn't gone the way he had hoped, and that we should wait it out. I left that phone call feeling physically sick. I tried to tell myself that there was nothing to worry about, all would be alright, and I decided there and then that whatever the outcome of the trade, I wanted to take whatever I had from the account and get out of the whole thing when the trade was done.

About a week later, he phoned me and said that we had made a loss on that trade, which honestly didn't surprise me at that stage. My gut instinct had finally kicked in, and I just wanted to get the heck out once and for all. I told him that I wanted out, but somehow, he managed to persuade me to put another £3000 in. Now I will definitely admit to being an odd bod, somewhat of a mis fit, but I never thought I was a stupid person, not until then that is. You see, these people that operate these scams really know how to manipulate people's emotions. They must honestly study the psychology of mind twisting. I could feel myself being controlled, but it was like I was someone else, not me being controlled. I can only imagine that the horror of what was going on with my consent didn't feel like it could be true. It didn't feel like it was actually me that this was happening to. So, I capitulated. The worst thing was that for some reason which I cannot now remember he wanted me to do the deposits in stages. So, whilst I was at work, I kept having to disappear up to the changing rooms to make the deposits, and each time I made a deposit, I had to fill in a wretched form! Sometimes I had to fill it more than once if they said my signature was not matching that on my bank card. So, I would go back down to work feeling so stressed and so anxious. But I couldn't let it show.

It was now late November 2018, and this was now the beginning of the real nightmare. Now I was 100% sure that I was the victim of a scam, and I just didn't know where to turn. I couldn't sleep, eat, or function properly. I couldn't tell anyone because I felt so ashamed at how stupid I'd been. I didn't think anyone could help, so I just kept hoping desperately that things would turn around in my favour. They didn't.

> **Early January 2019, he phoned me. He told me that things were not good, and that I should get a loan for £20,000...**

One Sunday in early January 2019, he phoned me. He told me that things were not good, and that I should get a loan for £20,000, put it into another crypto account and then there would be the leverage to do a big trade and come out on top. I felt like I was being led to my execution! We were on the phone for an hour. It took him that whole hour to persuade me. As I've mentioned, by then I knew it was scam, but by then I was also worn down, mentally, emotionally, even physically. He told me that I could repay it within the 14 days allowed to change your mind when taking out a loan. I think I just agreed to get him off the phone because I honestly felt like slitting my own throat. I really at that point understood what emotional torture felt like. So, I took the loan under his guidance on the desktop. It took about five days to be approved, and another couple of days to reach my bank account.

He was delighted and told me how to deposit the money in stages to this crypto currency exchange. He wanted to do it with me, but by that stage, something just snapped inside me. I'd had enough of this bloody man and his bloody crypto. I told him I would have to do it later as I was meeting my sister for lunch, which I actually was, and put my phone on silent. I went to my bank and stopped the pre-approval for the funds to go to the crypto exchange company. I had spoken to someone at the crypto exchange company who advised me that once the funds had been converted into crypto currency, they could not be converted back. I told him I didn't want to proceed and that I had been the unwitting victim of a scam. He was very kind. He told me to go to the bank to stop the pre-approval.

> I'd had enough of this bloody man and his bloody crypto...

I went and met my sister for lunch. At last, I felt some kind of peace within myself that at least I had seen sense and admitted to myself exactly what was going on before losing £20,000!!!

My phone rung constantly all afternoon, but I left it on silent. I knew who it was. Lunch went on for a few hours with my sister, and she never knew a thing about any of it.

Early next morning I phoned up the loan company and explained that I wanted to return the £20,000 and why. They were also very kind to me, and so I returned the money to them. At that point I was practically on my bended knees thanking God for his grace and wisdom, and his intervention to understand and admit my mistake and stop it there and then. My tears flowed, and I finally told my children and my two best friends, and then my sister.

The end of it all goes like this. A few days later, he phoned me. By now it was mid-January 2019. I cheerfully told him that I had paid back the loan of £20,000 to the loan company. He was delighted, that was until I told him what with! He thought I'd got the money from somewhere else to pay it back, and that I had in fact deposited the money into the crypto currency exchange. He assumed as he was aware of the pre-approval, that I had just gone ahead and done it. I have to say that although I do not believe in revenge, I could not help but feel some sense of justice when I heard the anger and frustration in his voice when I realised what I had done. His plan stumped, his control gone, his victim awoken and arisen from her slumber.

My bank returned the £6000 I had deposited into the company, once again there was me on bended knees sobbing my gratitude to the Lord God. I had not expected that! I had a few more phone calls from the crypto company, from the senior, senior accounts manager trying to lure me into the spider's web again. I shall not describe here the words I used on those calls. I will leave it to your imagination!

Why have I decided to share my story? I've always believed that people should be kind to one another, should lead with love, should seek ways to help one another, and reach out to protect one another. I want this message to be a warning, a loving reminder that if something looks too good to be true, then it absolutely is exactly that - it's a lie. I don't want to think of anyone going through the mental anguish that I went through, albeit a lesson I have well and truly learned. It's a lesson that almost cost me my sanity and could well have cost me my life.

DEDICATION
To my children - Matt, Heather, and Jordan; and to my big sister Belinda; and to my best friends Alan and Lorraine. Thank you for the love, understanding and support you showed me when I finally had the courage to tell you. Thank you for never judging me.

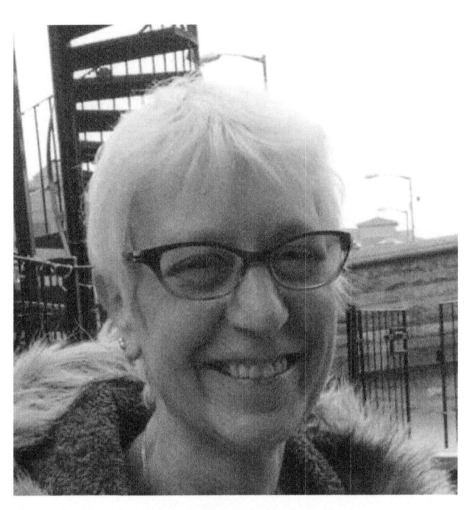

Caroline Brown

Caroline Brown

Caroline Brown is a 57 year old mother of 3 grown up amazing children, and has 5 beautiful grandchildren. Her most fulfilling job in the world of work were the 20+ years that she spent as a nurse.

She has always had a calling to help people, and still strives to do that now. At present, she works in retail, which gives her a roof over her head, but not a 'life'.

Caroline has, in recent months, felt a strong calling to deepen her understanding of, and strengthen her relationship with God, and now feels her calling is to help others to do the same in whatever way God wants instructs her to do.

She loves to travel, and has a goal of retiring somewhere hot, sunny, and near to the beach. Her motto is "You are not too old, and it's not too late", a message very dear to her heart.

Social Media Links:

Facebook: www.facebook.com/profile.php?id=100015289936467
LinkedIn: www.linkedin.com/caroline-brown-152b8a159
Instagram: www.instagram.com/cazbysea.cb

YouTube: https://www.youtube.com/channel/UCRqDrqwQRXFhBg7x-ZmkOwdw?view_as=public

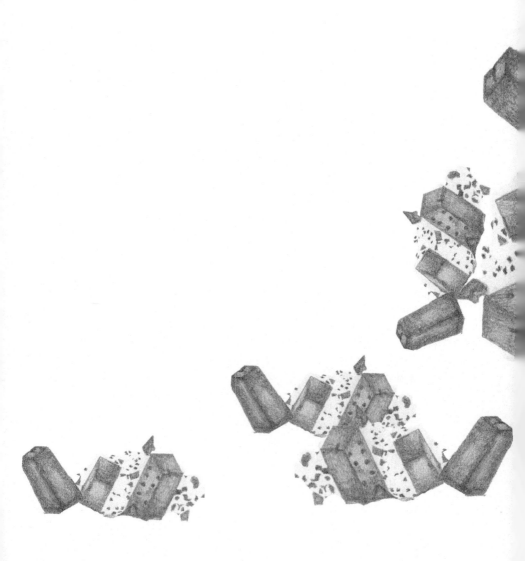

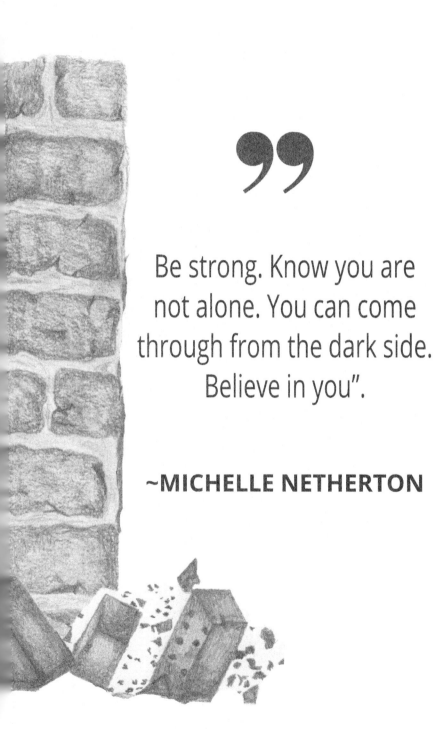

Be strong. Know you are not alone. You can come through from the dark side. Believe in you".

~MICHELLE NETHERTON

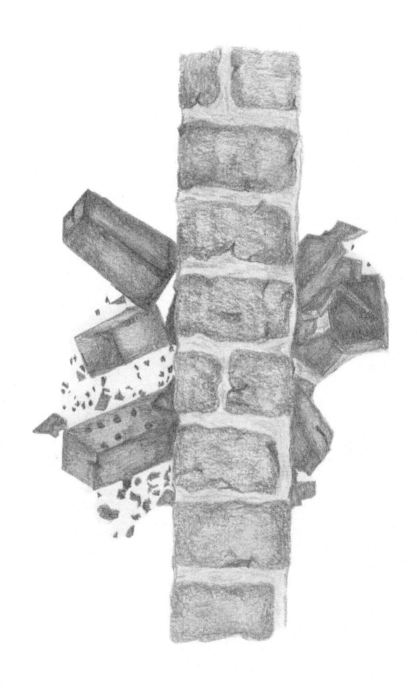

Up's & Down's of Parenthood

When you first find out you're pregnant you are filled with emotions of shock, joy, fear, expectation, amongst others.
I felt all of these...

I was 28 years old when I discovered I was pregnant with my first child, Jonah. I was mostly excited about the life growing within me. But I was fearful that maybe I wasn't ready to become a Mum and I asked myself the question of whether or not the father would stick around, as we'd only been dating 12 weeks and I was 6 weeks pregnant. He did stay and was more excited than me.

I had a relatively easy pregnancy, apart from the intense need for double cheeseburgers and having to have a glucose tolerance test. Things did go very smoothly, and I loved the feeling of my baby moving around and kicking. Then we got to the hard bit. I was woken up at 5:30am by a strange wetness in my bed. Half asleep, I shook Steve, my partner, awake and said, "I think I've wet myself", so he helped me up and as I got up, a wave of pain shook through my body and then the realisation hit me that the baby was coming.

I spent the next several hours timing contractions whilst playing cards with my mum, sister and Steve and so once they got to 5 minutes apart, we went to the hospital. As we got there, things started to slow again and then stop. So, the midwives hooked me up to an oxytocin drip to help things move quicker. It was a really long process, and I was totally exhausted after 24 hours, even with my mum, my sister and Steve there cheering me on. I was given some more medication to help me to rest and I don't really remember much about the next few hours, but I was told a few days later, that I was singing "the womble song" and telling everyone how much I loved them - even the nurses and mid-wives.

> Being naïve and so in love with my new-born baby, I believed them...

After over 41 hours and 30 minutes, we were finally nearly there. The baby got stuck so the midwife quickly put on a ventouse cup on Jonah's head and as she did, I contracted, but her hand slipped. Finally, he arrived and was placed in my arms. I knew then and there that I would do whatever I could, to encourage him in whatever he wanted to achieve in his life.

Because of the slip of the cup when he was born, Jonah had a 2-inch graze and dent to his skull, but I was told that it would correct itself as he grew. Being naïve and so in love with my new-born baby, I believed them. Unfortunately, I got postnatal depression after about 10 days when my milk dried up and I felt like a failure, so I just let my mum take over and feed him his formula whilst I retreated into myself.

I did start to do more things with Jonah - once the darkness of postnatal depression started to lift - and enjoyed watching him as he became more aware of his surroundings and started to smile, roll over and such like. After 6 months my partner Steve and I found a place of our own and moved with Jonah into a 2-bed flat.

Again, all seemed well. Jonah was developing really well and had started talking. He seemed to be excelling faster than I thought he would. By 10 months old he was a right little chatterbox and well ahead of where he should have been, but at 10 and a half months he just stopped.

Nothing came out of his mouth. He was completely silent. I voiced my concerns with Jonah's health visitor to which she replied, "You're a first-time mum. What do you know?!". It took me a while to regain my confidence because of what she had said to me, but after having no improvement with Jonah, I decided to teach him Makaton and I pushed to have a different health visitor.

Jonah had started sitting and staring at nothing, whilst rocking back and forth. He was physically hurting himself over silly things, e.g. when I told him he wasn't having ice cream for breakfast, which he signed to me, I was still told not to worry. I then started to do research online and so many times, the searches came back with AUTISM.

In all honesty, I didn't freak out too much. I just wanted to make sure that I got the right people involved to help with my son.

The questions do then start in your own head, "If all the things that I'm seeing on a daily basis was in fact not normal toddler be-haviour, could it be that he was starved of oxygen when being born as he got stuck? Did the ventouse cup on his head cause more damage than everyone said? or was I just being a "paranoid first-time mum" like the health visitor had said?". All these things were going through my head.

I did more and more research followed by attending many doc-tor's appointments, with me constantly telling them that some-thing wasn't right with my son and he needed to be referred to a paediatrician. I got pushed back so many times, but I refused to give up. Finally, after actually refusing to leave the doctors surgery until they referred him and sitting in there for 4 hours with Jonah running riot, they agreed and so our journey began.....

MICHELLE NETHERTON

A few months after Jonah's second birthday, I discovered that I was pregnant again and the fear I felt was horrible. Although I loved Jonah immensely, I feared there would be complications with this birth. I asked myself, "Would my second child have the difficulties that Jonah did? Would I be able to cope with a second child with these issues? Would Jonah cope with having a sibling? Would he hurt the baby as he hurt us and himself? I think that was when I decided to push professionals so much more because I knew my child needed help.

Shortly, after discovering I was pregnant, my big sister got really poorly and was rushed into hospital. They were unsure of what was going on and after a bit of pressure put on them, they finally conducted an MRI. They found a huge mass in my sister's brain and unfortunately, we were told it was cancer. It covered her whole frontal lobe, and it was a fast-growing tumour with a humongous name which we couldn't pronounce. So, she decided to call it "Neil" to make things easier and we all decided we wouldn't use the C word. Thankfully there were a few options for my sister and because she was well enough to make decisions, she decided on having half of the mass removed to give her a chance at it reducing with chemo after the surgery.

In the meantime, Jonah was getting better at communicating but I was still struggling on a daily basis, 9 weeks pregnant, and told the shocking news about my amazing sister. With the hormones racing in me and all the stress of daily life, I sunk into a depression and was put on antidepressants. All I saw for so long was darkness all around me. I knew that I was loved by my partner, Jonah and my other family members but some really dark thoughts passed through my mind in the following few weeks.

Things started to lighten though, with my first scan. Seeing that heartbeat inside of me shook me to the core. How could I be thinking such terrible things about my life, when this innocent life was growing inside me? Then and there, I decided to live everyday as the best I could. I was on this path for a reason and I was blessed to have a beautiful little boy, a loving partner and family. I needed to shake off the dark feelings and think of all the positives my future could bring.

Before long, my sister went into surgery. The wait then began and the fear of "would I ever see her again?" crept into my head. It was a very long wait but several hours later we were told it was a success. She was told that they couldn't remove all of it, but there was a possibility that with chemo it could shrink.

Not long after that, I had my second scan and found out we were having another boy. We were thrilled that he was healthy and was growing well. My sister started chemo but after a terrible couple of weeks decided to stop. Although we didn't really like her decision it was hers to make and we respected that her oncologist said she had to go and have an MRI every 3 months and they estimated that she would have 18 months left with us. My heart broke.

I had to have a second glucose tolerance test and found out I had gestational diabetes...

Fast forward a few more months and I was heavily pregnant and feeling very poorly. I had to have a second glucose tolerance test and found out I had gestational diabetes, so my cravings of pancakes with strawberries and cream were out of the window. And, because baby Rueben was measuring a few weeks ahead of what he should have been, the midwives decided that I shouldn't go past 38 weeks so was booked in for an induction. I was all set with my hospital bag, Jonah was with my mum and happy. I settled in for what could be a long process. Four hours later my lovely partner Steve came to the hospital with some lunch and that's when the pain in my back started. The midwives said that I was 3cm dilated, so Steve and I started walking around the hospital to try and move things along. It's then I received a phone call......

I broke down in tears as I learned from my cousin, that my Uncle had passed away and I was so gutted that I hadn't seen him the weekend before because I was tired. One of the many regrets in my life. Six hours later and totally exhausted, baby Rueben was born without any help from the midwives and was beautiful....

Jonah was nearly three by the time he actually saw the paediatrician and we only had a 20 minute appointment. I felt like all I did was talk about all the things that Jonah was doing - his lack of attention span, his constant frustration with himself, his aggressive behaviour how he'd basically destroyed our flat..... it just seemed to go on forever.

The paediatrician did a few tests and said that she was going to refer us to an occupational therapist and a speech and language therapist, and she would see us again in 6 months. So, it was more appointments and more waiting for answers and all the while our poor Jonah was struggling to communicate his needs at home and nursery and his behaviour was getting worse. There were some good things though as he finally said "Mum" again and my heart swelled with pride at every small achievement he made. He tried to like a new food and we would do a silent dance around the house because he didn't like loud noises. I felt that every day was a new learning experience with him. Yes, it was hard for Jonah, but it wasn't just Jonah who was struggling on a daily basis. I constantly felt like a bad mum because I got so overwhelmed with him, but he taught me so much.

> ## There it was in black and white - Jonah, my 4 year-old son, was on the autism spectrum...

Fast forward until just before Jonah's 4th birthday and we were back at the paediatricians. She said that she had all the reports from the other professional's, and they were ready to send all the evidence to the Autistic Spectrum Assessment Team. I felt a small sigh of relief.

Four months later the letter finally landed on my mat. Did I want to open it? This would change my son's life forever and this label would go everywhere with him. It took me a couple of hours before I opened it and there it was in black and white - Jonah, my 4 year-old son, was on the autism spectrum.

As a parent you feel so many emotions when you get that piece of paper with a diagnosis.

Relief that you've finally got somewhere from all the appointments and telephone conversations.
Grief because of the fear of what the future will hold for your child.
Sadness because you wanted so much for your child to be a high achiever and do so many things with their lives.
Determination to do whatever you can possibly do to be the voice for them and push whoever you have to, to get the provision in place for school so they won't struggle.

Along with Jonah's diagnosis of autism, the occupational therapist also diagnosed obsessive compulsive disorder and sensory processing disorder. As Jonah would soon be heading to primary school, the fight started to get what he needed put in place so he could attend a mainstream school. This is called an Educational Health Care Plan, and my goodness what a document that is! After 4 denials we were finally approved on the 5th time!

Meetings with the school started and it was decided that Jonah would have a staggered start into primary school. Because of all the change, we felt like this was the best option. I fell pregnant again and thankfully Jonah was finally in full time education so I could give more of my attention to my other two boys. School for Jonah was a complete and utter whirlwind with calls, early pickups because of overwhelm and much more I felt like my life was just about Jonah all the time and I felt that I couldn't be the mum I wanted to be to my boys because I was always talking to so many professionals all the time.

This was when I noticed that Rueben was struggling to catch his breath properly after running around at the park. So, I took him to the doctors, and they said that he could have juvenile asthma, so we started him on asthma pumps and things started to improve until he had to be blue lighted to hospital for having a cold. He was put on steroids and a nebulizer and after 24 hours of being in hospital, he was sent home with a further 5 days of steroids.

I think that's one of the horrible things about being a mum, when your child is so ill, that you can't get them to eat, you become helpless and will try them on any food. Little did we know that this wasn't the first time Rueben would have gastroenteritis and how much trouble we would have with his bowel and chest issues for the years to come.

Once Rueben was back on top form, we started him at a nursery near to Jonah's school. He absolutely loved it there but with being such a shy child, he did struggle with making friends and that's when we discovered that he had speech issues. I feel I should have realised there was an issue, but because I was constantly trying to be aware of what Jonah was doing, I was trying to protect Rueben and their younger brother Malachi, from Jonah's physical outbursts, it slipped through my filter, so Rueben was then referred to the speech and language therapist.

As Rueben was being referred to the paediatrician for his ongoing chest issue, Malachi (my third son) fell off of the trampoline to the floor and started having a seizure. He wasn't responding and his little body was still convulsing when the ambulance arrived. They couldn't get a response, so we were blue-lighted to the hospital and straight into resus. It took over 25 minutes for Malachi to come around. He finally squeezed my hand when I asked him to, and a huge relief washed over me. I can honestly say I've never been more scared in my whole life. I thought I was going to lose him. This was Malachi's first seizure which started our journey with epilepsy.

I can say that I have had a very stressful life so far with everything that's happened with my children. I love them all so much and even though we are going through some traumatic times I know that I am strong. And I want you to know that you are not alone and can come through from the dark side too. Believe in you.

DEDICATION

To all the SEN parents who are still fighting and to all who are winning the battle.

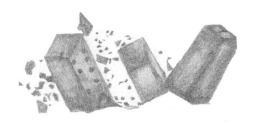

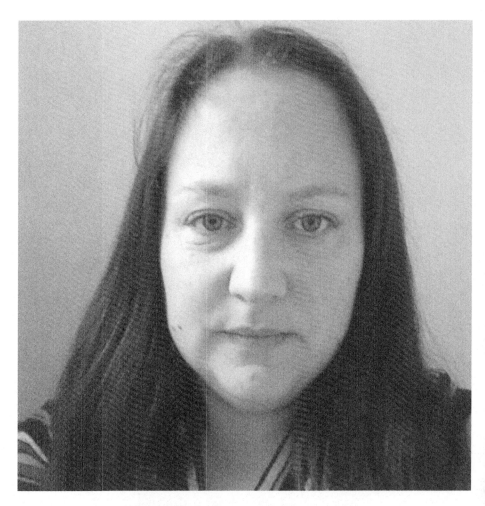

Michelle Netherton

Michelle Netherton

Michelle has diplomas in Autism Awareness, ADHD and Child Psychology. She is a Mum of 4 children (3 of which has Special Educational Needs). She lives in Cornwall, UK.

Michelle prides herself on learning as much as she can about the disabilities her children face and has a Child Care NVQ level 3 and is a qualified Senior Co-ordinator.

Her hobbies include going to the cinema, knitting, crocheting, reading, going for long walks and exploring with her children.

Social Media Links:

https://www.facebook.com/michelle.luff3

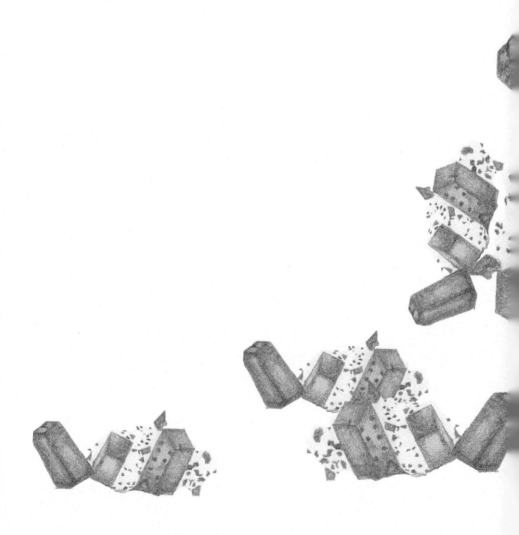

You are uniquely made
and are special.
You can change the
world".

~LOUISA MOULTON

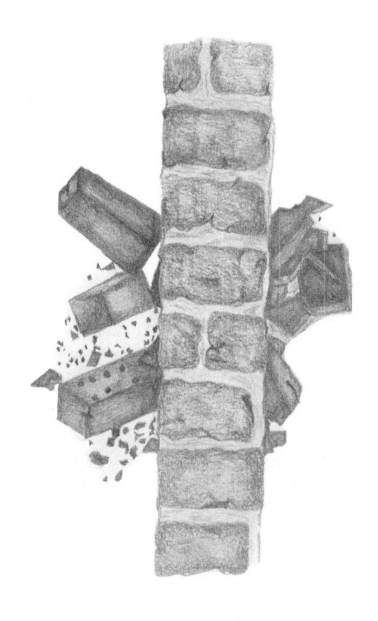

From Struggles To Success!

I was diagnosed at the age of 7 with Autism Asperger's Syndrome. It was very difficult to process as I was just in my early stages of learning and getting to know what being a child was all about...

Everything I was thinking and feeling, up to that point, was natural for me and then to be given this news and having to adapt to my family's thoughts of "don't teach everything to Louisa at home and don't give her any mainstream or high-level education" was enough to make you angry, sad and upset.

I wanted to grow, learn, expand and be independent like everyone else. I could do it!

My parents wanted other people to keep an eye on me, so they sent me to 2 respite care centres near to where I lived. I'd meet people in wheelchairs and with other special needs and disabilities who were more unable than me. I would sometimes stay overnight and experience different things too (some not so good) and on different occasions I would be in difficult situations where some staff would be loud and cross with some people too. Overall, it was nice, but I felt that the environment wasn't a good place for me to be. I took lots from the respite centres for when I grew older like looking at how people behave and interact and also to learn more about the traits of Autism. My biggest thing was and still is to try to prove to others that I'm completely different to the claims of how some people behave while having Autism.

From the age of 12, my parents sent me to special needs boarding schools, and I stayed at the first one for 5 years. It started off okay, but I was halfway through my 5 years at that school when I started to be bullied during the day and also when living in the boarding accommodation too. I wasn't coping well at all. I felt sad, upset and didn't know who to talk to or where to turn. I felt isolated.

> **In the church you're accepted. At school and home, I was surrounded by non-stop judgement and negativity...**

I wasn't coping at home either. So, when I did go home, I had some help from a very kind neighbour called Helen. From the age of 6 she had watched over me a lot as our gardens were next to each other. She invited me to join her at church and I started to experience the church in a fun way. She showed me the Bible, taught me about Christianity and asked if I would like to attend Sunday School. I said yes as I felt it played a big part in me coping and finding the strength to not feel useless or be different to others. In the church you're accepted. At school and home, I was surrounded by non-stop judgement and negativity. Which in a simplified way, I felt was mostly what my family looked at me like for the first 17 years of my life, and so having this very kind neighbour Helen helping me loads while I was growing up meant a lot. I am so grateful to her.

I was bullied at my first boarding school and treated unfairly because I made a mistake. It was a small silly thing I did without thinking – as I'm sure you may have made mistakes yourself – I'm going to share with you what I did.

Without thinking of the consequences, I took some money, a few coins, from a pot or bag which was by my mum's bedside at home. She reported what I did to the caretaker of the school and so after that everyone was keeping an eye on me. They would call me names, be nasty to me and send me horrible messages like "You are the most bad behaving girl in the school!" More things happened, which I don't want to share but it's not an experience that I liked at all. And I thought; "Here comes a big test to coping with unfair people who only know you a little bit, but still, when just hearing rumours about you they decide to suddenly bully and scare you". That awful experience is something I can never forget – things like that stay with you for life. It was the first most difficult 5 years in school I had in my education.

As I was regularly given the "here comes the bad girl" message and other people said "don't trust her whatever you do" it really hurt – the looks, stares, pointing and words being whispered. In the evenings the staff checked up on me and had a chat with me regularly telling me that they would be keeping an eye on me.

Going to sleep of a night-time I had fearful thoughts on what the next day would bring, how nasty people were going to be and what they would say. I decided to play music on my Walkman to help me relax and go to sleep. It helped to have less fears and to be calm. It also helped me, as I listened to the music to know that I am strong, and I found I was able to sleep better. With doing that, I was able to think that if trouble occurred, I could just try and not take it too hard - whatever people say about me or do – I am strong and I will be okay.

People checked on me, had chats and I also wrote lots of notes too. The moments when things were tough, I talked with my friend Helen about my issues, and she helped me and reminded me that I'm a winning person and that I am going to succeed in lots of new stuff that I'll be doing after having completed all of my education. If she talked to my mum, she would say to my mum that she has an amazing daughter who is more able and ready than she thinks and that she'd be impressed when she sees how much I had developed.

I changed boarding schools, so I was further away from home and this one was a bit better for what I got while being there. The students and staff were a bit better in being fun, kind and supportive to each other. I settled, felt comfortable and relaxed as I wasn't being bullied either. I learned a lot more and slowly thought; "Here comes my chance to work hard, to be even more clever and to show people that even though I have Autism, I can still do well".

> **It felt amazing! I showed them how clever I was and how I could set goals...**

I slowly but surely began to show how much I could do. It felt amazing! I showed them how clever I was and how I could set goals. I reminded myself every day what it was I wanted and needed and went for it. I felt so proud of myself.

While I was at that second boarding school, my mum and dad decided to get a divorce because they both weren't very good together. I saw when I was at home with them that they were very argumentative a lot, didn't like the same interests or do loads together. They preferred to be apart than together, so this news didn't get to me too much.

I remember on one birthday at the boarding school, my mum bought me an autobiography of Lord Sugar. This inspired me to finish my education, start my own venture and be self-employed by running my own business. So, after I finished my second boarding school, I went to a special needs boarding college and it was my favourite place of all time.

I went to that boarding school feeling very positive because I knew exactly what I wanted to do when I left, after having read Lord Sugar's book, thanks to my mum. At the college I learned a lot of real workplace skills (retail and office). I also learned a lot of independent living skills too that I could use away from home so that they can help me to live independently.

After leaving the special needs college, my life was controlled by the system of where I lived, what I did and how I would get money to pay for my things. It felt like I had no control or say at all. I moved into supported living and went onto benefits. I lived in a communal place and volunteered at a local Cancer Research charity shop, which was a fun activity which I enjoyed doing.

I've moved quite a lot and met so many new friends and achieved lots of skills too. Richard, a friend I met 2 years ago, has shared with me his experience of Autism and it's great having someone to talk to and share things with. He has also played a big part in helping me get started and learn about a new type of work connected to my goal to be self-employed. I am now slowly learning and doing this, which is network marketing.

Over the years I have been treated appallingly. Sometimes I have felt that no-one listens to me or takes my opinions into consideration, especially as it's my life. I've been unfairly looked at for far too long and I know that I deserve more. I've missed out on looking for work and earning money rather than being on benefits, but I have thought of how kind some people have been, and I am grateful for those people who have helped me over the years.

I know I have Autism, but I have also goals that I am aiming for and I want a life full of fun and happiness. I have achieved a lot and each time I do, I smile. It's a great feeling!

Learning new skills and helping other people with Autism to know that they can have the traits of being on the spectrum, but they are uniquely made and are special too is a goal of mine. They need to know that they can change the world, as I am going to.

LOUISA MOULTON

DEDICATION

I am dedicating this chapter to Richard Fey. Thank you for everything you have done and constantly do to help me.

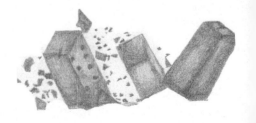

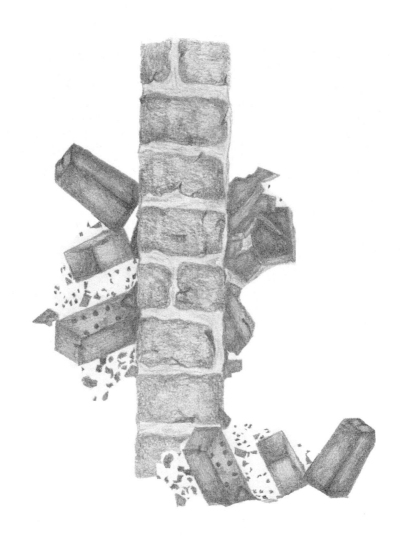

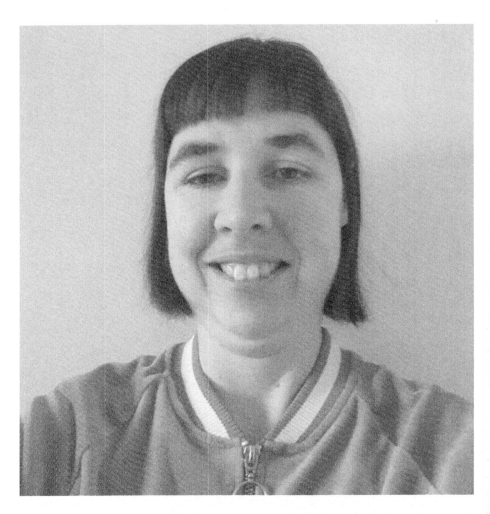

Louisa Moulton

Louisa Moulton

Louisa is a Network Marketing Professional based in the UK. She is an Autism Advocate after being diagnosed with Autism at 6yrs old.

She is ambitious and aspirational and has a lot to give and share on this interview. She is showing people that they can accomplish anything, and not to allow your special needs to hold you back. She loves reading, listening to music, having fun and economics.

CONNECT WITH LOUISA HERE:
Facebook: https://www.facebook.com/louisa.moulton.7
Shop with Louisa : https://www.avon.uk.com/store/louisa-m/
FB page: https://www.facebook.com/Lm-wellness-386156498777344

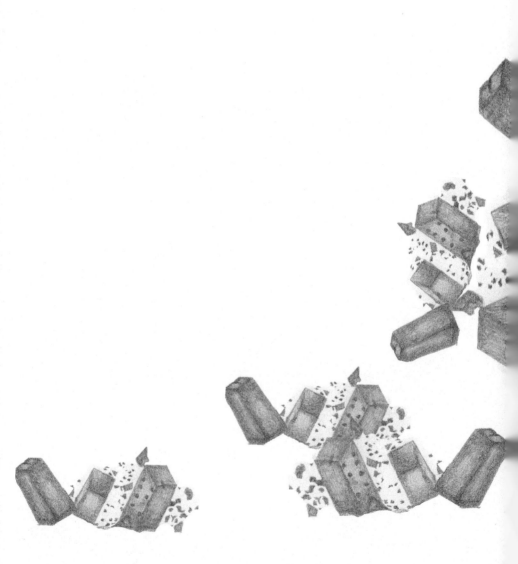

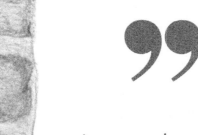

Accept that you are loved and you are enough".

~**LORRAINE FORD**

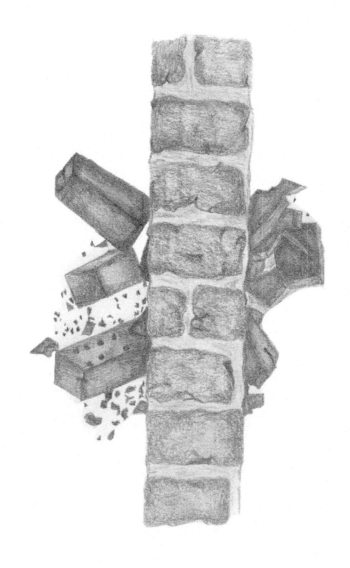

Life can Change in an Instant

I was 18 years old, and I had just got engaged to the boy I had been dating since I was 14.
I was working in a bank, had my own car and I was enjoying life to the full.
Plenty of friends, plenty of parties, aerobics classes, walking, playing in a brass band and generally having fun.

I t was December, always a really busy time at work, but it was a fun time with excited customers and Christmas cheer in abundance. I had a bout of flu, and went back to work, with less energy and enthusiasm than usual but I carried on.

Friday night arrived, and feeling shattered, I went home. Having previously arranged with a friend to go for drinks in town, I kept to the arrangement, so as not to let her down, but I didn't feel much like going, I was so tired...

We caught the bus from her house and headed into town. It was heaving! The world and his wife were out having Christmas drinks! I started to feel really poorly. I didn't want to drink, and the noise and bustle was making me feel uneasy.

LORRAINE FORD

To be honest, I just wanted to go home. But having caught the bus, this wasn't an option. The evening finally ended, and we ran for the last bus. I don't remember any more of the journey and I don't remember going to bed.

> I just remember waking up in someone else's house, with numb legs, tingling arms, unable to breathe, and feeling very sick...

I just remember waking up in someone else's house, with numb legs, tingling arms, unable to breathe, and feeling very sick. It was the strangest, weirdest feeling I had EVER had, and I didn't like it. I didn't like it at all!

I managed to drive myself home in the morning and collapsed in the door. My Mum helped me to bed. From that moment on, my life changed... My sparkle had gone. I was exhausted – All the time!

I don't mean like you are when you have had a really busy day and it's getting near to bedtime... I mean exhausted to the point of hysteria, shaking, feeling sick, arms and legs like lead, too heavy to move exhausted. I didn't feel right, and it didn't feel right. Something was off and most definitely wrong!

My body hurt, my muscles ached right through to the bone, and my bones hurt. The best way I can describe it is like the pain and exhaustion you feel when you have the flu...total lethargy. I was unable to hold a book up to read, sometimes I couldn't even lift my head from the pillow. I was light and noise sensitive and the ability to concentrate to read or watch a film became a distant memory.

I couldn't control my body temperature. Even in the height of summer I had a hot water bottle and a duvet. I slept with a bucket by my bed because of the overwhelming nausea.   Clothes hurt, brushing my hair hurt, I could just about crawl to the toilet. Bathing and showering would take the little bit of energy I had gathered.

The most annoying thing I found was that no two days were the same. I couldn't understand it! The symptoms were the same, just to varying degrees. I was always tired, and I was always in pain. Some days I could go to work, some days I couldn't physically get out of bed. Some days I was able to go out after work, and some days I couldn't. The unreliability of what my body was doing to me was becoming a serious issue.

My mental health was starting to deteriorate. One minute I was happy, the next crying uncontrollably. I wanted to be left alone, but then complained that no one was with me. I gave up playing in the band. I gave up my exercise classes and going for walks. Going to work was all I could manage, if that. I had started having to cancel plans with friends, and eventually those friends became more and more distant, and I became more and more isolated.

I kept going to the doctors. I could hear myself saying things like; "I just feel really ill", "I am so tired". I felt pathetic, who goes to the doctor's because they are tired? It was so upsetting.

That was when my whole world came tumbling down around me as I was diagnosed with post viral fatigue syndrome and then M.E./CFS (Myalgic Encephalomyelitis/Chronic Fatigue Syndrome).
My thoughts were "What do I do now? How will I live my life? How will I achieve my dreams? I want children!". Such a lot to get my head around!

I was put on so many tablets and medications, just to get me to function throughout the day - I felt like I was rattling! I was existing, but not living.

I got married and moved about 20miles away from my parent's house and the bank where I worked. I was living on a farm, 3 miles from the outskirts of a tiny village in the middle of nowhere.

LORRAINE FORD

I struggled into work as much as I could. One week I would manage the whole week. The next, just a couple of days. There was no pattern to it, and because when I was there, I was walking and talking to customers and work colleagues, seemingly with no issues, people seemed to doubt I was telling the truth and was skiving. Even though I had a doctor's note for every time I was off, people from work started to telephone me when I was off. I knew it was work, because I could hear the office, the customers and staff talking in the background, although no one spoke to me. I would often get three to four calls a day.

One thing that really got to me was the fact that there was another girl, who would go raving every weekend, would call in sick on a Monday because she felt ill, and the staff sent her flowers for being poorly! Can you imagine how that made me feel?

> **Yet I was being made to feel like the fraudster! The way I was treated still hurts to this day...**

I was genuinely ill, with a doctor's note, and she was having withdrawal symptoms from popping E's! Entirely her choice and in her control. Yet I was being made to feel like the fraudster! The way I was treated still hurts to this day. I felt so ill and in pain ALL the time and being made to feel as though I was making it up. It was heart-breaking.

I was so poorly, I couldn't even put a shovel of coal on the fire to keep the place warm, let alone cook, clean and do the normal stuff people do on top of a fulltime job. My 'good days' were painful, and a huge struggle, but I learned to paint a smile on and carried on, best I could, even though inside I was falling apart - physically as well as mentally.

Have you ever experienced this? The weight of putting on a brave face, coupled with not wanting to let everyone down started to overwhelm me. I was a failure, useless, a burden to everyone.

One day I sat in the lunchroom, just gazing at the prescription I had just collected. There were so many high dosage pills in my hands...if only I was brave enough to take them, it would all stop. A colleague came in, interrupted my train of thought and I carried on again. Still feeling a burden, still feeling a failure, but still alive... for now.

My Mum was then diagnosed with breast cancer, my marriage was more a friendship than a marriage and I was on more and more medication feeling totally out of control of every aspect of my life. My husband and I agreed to separate, although amicable in the end, it had been a mentally abusive relationship at times, and I, once again, felt like a failure. That I had let everyone down in not making it work. I moved back to the village I was brought up in, my younger brother and my parents were still there, and I had some support around me again.

I bought my own place - a mobile home, 40x10. Very different to a 3-bedroom farmhouse, but it was mine and I loved it. I started afresh.

I was what they call a 'high functioning depressive' - to the outside world I had everything. My own place, a car, a good job, family close by, but behind closed doors it was a different story.

I was broken.

Mentally I was broken.
Emotionally I was broken.

I had good days and bad, good months and bad. Never a pattern, just going through the motions, feeling like I was wading through mud or walking up a sand hill. Keeping on going but never getting anywhere. Never understanding what I had done that was so wrong, to make my life this way.

I was then made redundant!

Questions like; "Why was I never good enough? What was wrong with me? I do my very best for everyone, in every way, why was it never enough?".

LORRAINE FORD

I knew no matter how I felt that I needed a job. I had bills to pay, and I was on my own. I only had myself to rely on. I went for an interview. I got the job! I Loved it! I entered a phase of relative wellness and was able to do a little more, and whilst on a day out with some friends, I met and immediately fell for the man who was to become my second husband.

I still had severe anxiety and depression, but as usual, I kept it all hidden. I still went out of my way to be as helpful as I could to people, no matter how I was feeling on the inside. Maybe people just thought I was ok...

I wasn't. I was dealing with a whole heap of physical and mental challenges every day.

Pain and exhaustion overwhelmed me once again. Soon I was back having more and more time off work and in the end the doctor signed me off work completely. Now I felt really useless!

I had 2 ectopic pregnancies. I couldn't even do that right! The questions and self-loathing started creeping into my head again. Having a baby was all I had ever really wanted, and now that chance had been ripped away from me too! My husband had an affair and left. Another failure.

At the ripe old age of 34 I was becoming resigned to the fact that I wasn't good enough to be a wife, and a mother and fate was showing me this in no uncertain terms. The life I had dreamed of was like a cruel nightmare being played out in front of me by everyone else I knew. Everyone except me was happily married, was a parent, was healthy and I felt like I was sat on the sidelines watching - physically and mentally ill, with no job, no income, no children and 2 failed marriages.

Was I ever going to be healthy and happy?
How would I meet someone? Who would want me anyway? I wasn't exactly a catch!

All of the self-doubt kicked in and started to overload my brain. The derogative words and sentences kept repeating in my head. I kept going over and over everything that had happened, instead of looking at all the good that I had actually achieved.

Weirdly, in the midst of all this I took a turn for the better. A neighbour who I had known for about 10 years, and had always looked out for me, and I him and he started looking out for me a bit more. He did a few little jobs that I had been left with and we became close. It was wonderful, as we were friends, and he knew my history. Before we knew it love had blossomed. It was great. We had both wanted children in our lives, but both thought that our chances had passed us by until we started talking.

He thought it was too late for him because of his age. And because of my history, we thought it would be impossible for me to conceive naturally and that IVF would be my only option. Was this something he was willing to consider? It Was! We came to the conclusion that maybe this was what we had both been waiting for. The right set of circumstances with the right person. We went for IVF and were successful 1st time! It was meant to be!

Negative thoughts crept in occasionally throughout the pregnancy; "Was I good enough? How would I cope with a baby? I wasn't worthy of being happy" etc etc..... especially when I ran into some complications and there was a high risk of us losing the precious cargo I was carrying.

Our daughter Abby was born by elective C-section (because of my CFS it was decided to be the safer option) weighing in at 5lb14oz. Our tiny precious miracle was here, and we were ecstatic.

I secretly decided that even if my mental health took a turn for the worse afterwards, I wouldn't tell anyone except my mum. Because of my mental health history, I was so scared they would take our baby away. Fortunately, I didn't have another depression episode for a few years.

I was over the moon, everything seemed to be going right – my CFS was under control and aside from normal new mum anxiety everything was going well. Then we were given the devastating news that my Dad had oesophageal cancer. It was terminal. He died holding his beloved granddaughter, who had reached the ripe old age of 7 months! My heart was broken, but I had Abby and my Mum, and they were both relying on me...

Sometime later, Abby had to have a heart operation, all went well, and she started school. I threw myself into getting involved

LORRAINE FORD

and helping wherever and whenever I could. I became a TA and a lunchtime supervisor, and I loved it, but I became really ill again and spent days at a time in bed. I had to give up working again and my Mum took an active role in our lives, taking Abby to and from school, and looking after her and me until my partner got home from work. Mum was then diagnosed with cancer for the 2nd time and had to undergo chemo.

I was too ill to help her and so as I lay there in bed the questions started to creep into my head again; "Why was I so useless?".

Instead of me being there for her, most of the time it was the other way around. She stayed strong and kept me together, even talking me through panic attacks on the phone because she was unable to have contact with anyone during her treatment. 5 years later she died, unexpectedly. I kept going. I had to.

I had lost my support network and remember all those people I helped when I was poorly? Well, not one of them stepped up for me! Shocking really when you think about it. I am a nice kind and wonderful person who would do anything for anyone and yet no-one thought I was important enough to even ask how we were all doing! No-one even offered to do the school run for me and I didn't want to ask in case the school got involved and they took Abby - the stigma of mental health and invisible illness and not being able to cope is very scary. I sank into deep depression, my head told me yet again, that I clearly didn't matter or mean a thing to anyone.
On New Year's Day 2019, in the middle of a family day out, I ended up on a notorious cliff. What was the point? No-one cared and I wasn't worth the space I took up on the planet. I was a waste of oxygen. I couldn't manage to cook a full meal and I could barely do any housework. Abby would cook, clean, put the washing on, put the shopping away and do all the things I was meant to do for her and her Dad.

 Abby was in primary school. Her Dad was working a fulltime phys-ical job and they were both coming home to be a carer for me. I wasn't needed...they would be better off without me.
Thankfully, they were there, and they took me home.
Something within me changed from that moment...

I decided once and for all I needed to sort this out. I couldn't do anything about my M.E. or my energy levels, but I could work on my mindset and sort my head out.

I referred myself to the local mental health team. I started another course of CBT. It actually made a lot more sense this time around, and I was willing to do anything it took. Slowly I started to feel a little brighter and I got some healing too. I had never done this before. I didn't think I was worthy of spending the money on me, but my other half assured me I was worth it, and I am So glad I did! My whole central nervous system was out of sync from spending the last 30 years on high alert, super sensitive to everything, and now things were starting to realign, I was Amazed!

I took my gratitude practice much more seriously. I started working on my mindset to turn the negative thoughts around quicker. I have found peace by reducing the negativity and watching my circle. I still have very bad days, but I am so much better at controlling the fall out now. I have even been able to reduce my meds!

The only downside at the moment is the physical side of my invisible illness, but I am learning to live with it better and accept it after all these years. I am actually grateful for it because it has allowed me to take life at a slower pace and enabled my daughter to be a competent, caring and empathic young person.

I used to be angry that she should have to do such 'grown up stuff' and that I should be doing it and not her, but she will be a wonderful adult, and I am blessed to have her and my partner looking after me. I am thankful to be able to come to terms with and accept that I am loved for me, and that I am enough.

DEDICATION

I dedicate this chapter to my beautiful daughter Abby. Thank you for being an amazing Light in my life. You are Loved more than you could ever imagine.

I also dedicate this chapter to my wonderful partner Grip for all that you do. You are truly a blessing. AAF xx

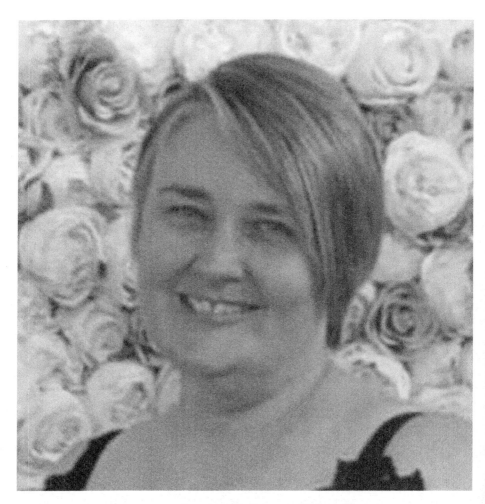

Lorraine Ford

Lorraine Ford

Lorraine Ford is a Mum to a 12-year old daughter called Abby. She is in Network Marketing focusing on Health and Wellness.
She is also a Part-time Courier and has CFS / ME and has battled anxiety and depression for over 30yrs.
Lorraine's goal is to help people feel better about themselves and for them to know they are not alone.
She played in a brass band for 30yrs and has also FIRE-WALKED!!!

Social Media Links:
Facebook: https://www.facebook.com/phoenixdiamonds

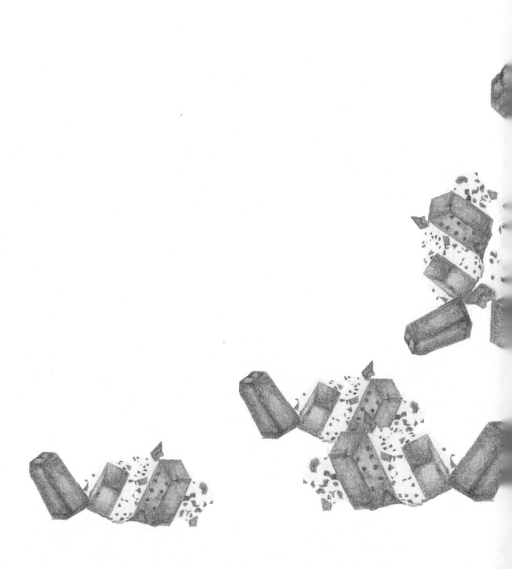

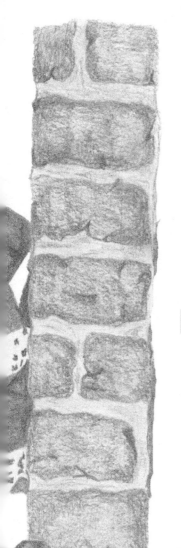

99

Before making a
connection with a
human being, get to
know yourself first and
then your partner".

~LAKEISHA McGEE

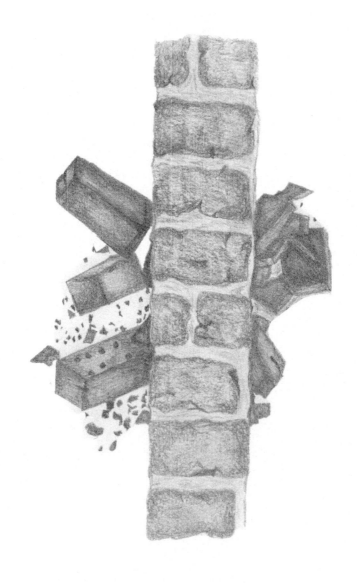

SURVIVING THE UNEXPECTED

*Survivor "a person who survives,
especially a person remaining alive after an event in
which others have died; a person who copes well with
difficulties in their life".*

I've always been studious, a hard worker, competitive and determined to win. Whatever I set my mind to do, I do it! Growing up my parents expected me to do better than they did and the expectation was for me to go away to college. Now I had never seen anyone in my family actually go away to college as I'm one of the oldest grandchildren on both sides, but it was my goal. I wanted to go to Grambling University and live in the sorority house. I ran track and was pretty darn good at it. Grambling had offered me a scholarship. What a dream it seemed like that would be and I almost made it. It was my senior year in high school and I had transferred to Plano East Senior High School, in Plano Texas, to live with my biological father, something I'd never done before. The previous summer had brought turbulence between my parents and I somehow thought I knew more than they did.

My parents were great parents (my mom & paw-paw). I had everything I wanted and needed, including my own car. I wanted more independence and felt I was mature enough to make my own decisions because I was a senior. My parents gave me an alternative;

follow the rules or move with my biological father. I called their bluff and they sent me on my way. I will never forget the pain I caused my mom. She felt so betrayed, hurt and she didn't deserve it. All the hard work she had done and she wouldn't be able to experience the fruits of her labor. The joy of seeing me go to prom, the reward of me just graduating, and her being able to be apart of all my senior activities. I'm her only child and we were best friends. I now know how selfish I was. At the time, I was in honors classes doing well and running track, so transferring schools would throw it all away because I couldn't join the team at the new school considering I had missed tryouts. I didn't care. I had a point to prove, so I left.

> "If I could go back and tell my 17 year old self a few things, I would surely tell her to slow down and take your time and get to know a person...

Moving in with my biological father wasn't better, it was just a different set of circumstances. My dad had a new family. I had three younger siblings which made it hard. I wasn't used to sharing and I really wanted to develop a better relationship with my dad but it didn't seem as if it was going to happen. I had spent some time with my other family in the summers but never had I lived with them. I enjoyed living with my dad but the expectations, rules, and lack of material things were overwhelming to a spoiled only child, needless to say it only lasted three months and back to Chicago I went.

It was around November 1991 when I returned home and it felt great. My parents and I agreed upon some new normals and began to put our family back together. One weekend, I went to a party with some friends and I met this young man. I had never seen him before and he intrigued me. He had on dress pants and a buttoned up shirt, attracting me to what I thought represented sophistication. I didn't know much about him but I was sprung and I was going to get to know him. I was 17 and so naive. I had only one puppy love relationship before this which ended in pain, lies and deceit.

We began to hang out, he was 21 at the time. I still didn't know him and honestly because I was so green, I didn't even really know what to expect in a relationship with a young man and not one that was more mature than I. If I could go back and tell my 17 year old self a few things, I would surely tell her to slow down and take your time and get to know a person. J was a kind person and came from a good family but was into a lot of mischief that I hadn't been exposed to. I was truly a free spirit, but my parents really had sheltered me so I lacked experience and examples. The relationship progressed, not sure what he thought we were but I thought we were a couple. Fast forward a few months down the line to the first time we became intimate, I remember exactly where and what date it was: January 20th, my moms birthday.

February 1992 rolls around my senior year three months away from graduation after a track meet I wasn't feeling like myself. I didn't even think about pregnancy. Yes, I had unprotected sex and I wasn't on birth control but we had only done it once. My mother had always said when you're ready let me know. Well, I hadn't planned on being ready that soon I had begun to feel very tired after track meets and practice. I had never felt like this before, my boobs were sore and I was scared so I took a pregnancy test. The home pregnancy test came back positive. I could not believe it, so I took another one. My friend, who would become my son's godmother, Gina was there. I didn't know what to do, how could this happen? We had only had sex one time, what was I going to do?

When I told J I was pregnant he basically said whatever I wanted to do he would support. Little did I know there had been another girl who had an abortion a few months prior and I would soon find out that he was a cheater with more girls saying they too were pregnant. If I had known these things, I'm not sure if I would've made the same choices. One of the hardest things i'd ever had to do was tell my parents that I had failed them and to know that I had disappointed them, broke me. Let me explain; I didn't meet my biological father until I was seven. He was incarcerated all that

LAKEISHA McGEE

time and my mother never took me to see him. A year or so later, my mom married my paw-paw (step-father). I rejected him in the beginning because I had just met my biological father and was trying to establish a relationship with him. I was confused and I was a kid.

Over the years paw-paw and I became very close. He was a great father: he never missed parent conferences, cooked for me, brought me turtles home every night from work, came to every track meet, he loved me. Paw-paw had five sons but I was the daughter he always wanted, his only daughter and he spoiled me. We had worked so hard to get to this place, so to disappoint him hurt me so much. There were several of my acquaintances in the community that had become pregnant and I remember my paw-paw saying he was so glad it wasn't me. Keep in mind I'm three months away from high school graduation.

 It's funny how parents know you. My mom knew I was pregnant before I told her. We cried together and although she was disappointed, she was supportive as always. I don't remember how we told Paw-Paw but what I can say is that I broke his heart and those next nine months were hell. He didn't talk to me the whole time I was pregnant. He couldn't even look at me. When we did talk, it was an argument and it was horrible. I am the woman that I am today because of my dad. He poured into me; making sure I was secure, had great self esteem and I knew my worth. I had destroyed a relationship that took years to build.

My pregnancy was stressful. I was embarrassed, confused and lord knows I'm inexperienced.

 J was young and not really prepared to be a father. He tried, but his support was inconsistent and unreliable. He made it to some Dr. Appointments with me but not nearly enough. He was told if he wasn't there when our son was born, he wouldn't have his name but unbeknownst to me, he was still cheating and it appeared that I was preparing to be a single parent. I had no clue what was about to happen and I was unsure if I wanted to be a parent. I was stressed to the max!

I remember going into my moms room. She was laying down so I got in the bed and laid beside her. We talked about all of my options but the only alternative I considered was abortion. I come from a family that doesn't believe in terminating pregnancies and my mother expressed that, but she also said she would support my decision. She said "Today is the only day we will have this discussion. Once you decide, that's what we're doing." Obviously, we never had that talk again.

When bringing a child into this world, my advice for you is to take time and get to know the person because having a child is a lifetime commitment. I see this way too often, parents bringing children into this world without even knowing the other partner's last name and furthermore, not even knowing themselves. As an only child, I feel that I had always been mature but preparing to be a parent changed my life and made me grow up overnight.

> **She said "Today is the only day we will have this discussion. Once you decide, that's what we're doing." Obviously, we never had that talk again...**

November 2nd, I was walking around inside of Burlington with my mom and I began to cramp. I felt this wet gush in my panties, which later I found out was my mucus plug. My mom and I went to the bathroom and she confirmed that it was indeed my mucus plug and that I was probably in labor. We walked home, and by the time I got there the cramps had intensified. I couldn't go any further than the garage, so I just lay there in the middle of the floor in a fetal position. My mom called my doctor and they instructed her to perform some breathing exercises with me. A few hours passed by and the cramps got worse. The pain was unbearable and so I knew it was time to go to the hospital. My brother Ronnie took me to the hospital where they admitted me because I was, indeed, in labor.

LAKEISHA McGEE

My labor lasted 28 hours and in the middle of pushing, I began to regurgitate. Something was wrong. My mom panicked and I was in and out of consciousness. I hear her yell to the doctors, "Save my baby, I don't know that other baby." I honestly don't remember what happened from there, but in some kind of way they had gotten everything under control. I was delirious when it was all said and done. My parents, brother and his girlfriend, and finally J and his mom were all in attendance. Although J was late, as a first time parent, I was happy we were both there to experience our child being born. I gave birth to a 5 pound, 6 ounces, 14 inches long healthy baby boy. Our lives changed on that day, and once my son was born, me and my dad's relationship began to mend immediately.

> "
> Aside from him lying and cheating, he still wasn't ready to accept his role in being a father. I began to not feel myself...

Over the next few months, I focused on being a mom, and adjusting to college which began that spring commuting back and forth. Throughout this time, I was experiencing a lot of turmoil with J. Aside from him lying and cheating, he still wasn't ready to accept his role in being a father. I began to not feel myself. I had a lack of energy and was no longer excited about life. I later learned that I had postpartum depression, which my doctor never explained to me that this could possibly occur. It was bad. I flunked out of school the first semester because everything just became way too much.

Paw-paw came to withdraw me from school and again, I had disappointed him. I felt horrible.

I thank God for overcoming my postpartum depression because that same year I was experiencing that at 18, a 36 year old African American prominent doctor, jumped from her penthouse home in downtown Chicago, over the exact same thing. My parents and I agreed that it was best I took time off from school and instead got a job. I worked at the post office and after a few months, I was able to buy myself a brand new car and was working on getting my own apartment. I always felt like once you had a child, you were grown and needed your own space. I started going out more, meeting new people, and was still back and forth with J. We were trying to coparent the best way we knew how but it was toxic because one day we were together and the next broken up.

I was in the shower one day, and my mom came in the bathroom looked at me, and told me I was pregnant. I immediately denied the allegations because there was no way. A few weeks later, it was confirmed that I was. This time, my pregnancy was different. After I found out I was pregnant, a month later I moved out and was on my own. I was pregnant again and I had a 1 and a half year old. J had left and went back to college and was living his life. I worked at the post office as long as I could and my son was going to daycare. I commuted between Elgin, Shaumburg and Carol Stream everyday. The stress alone from doing that, damn near killed me. The manual labor from my job became too much and I resigned. I started working at a temp company, which was sweet, being that it was only two exits away from my apartment, only I still had to travel to Shaumburg to drop my baby off at daycare and then travel all the way back to where I lived for work. I was exhausted and depressed every single day. My mom came to stay with me so that I wouldn't be alone as it got closer time for me to give birth.

I woke up one morning and was cramping really bad. I saw that my plug had came out and was in a lot of pain. For some reason, I didn't want to go to the hospital but as the pain progressed, 3 hours later me and my mom go to the hospital. This baby didn't take any time to come. By the time I got to the hospital, his head was already crowning. By the time mom put on her scrubs, he was halfway out. He was 7 pounds, 14 ounces and 16 inches long. A couple days later I was home and the boys paternal grandmother picked up my first son to keep him a few days. At that moment, I realized shit had just got real real for me. I had two kids, with no college education. What was I going to do?

I enrolled at Elgin Community College and began to work hard at being successful. School had always been easy for me but now I was a non-traditional student juggling parenting two children. I needed support. I worked, I went to school, and I raised my sons.

LAKEISHA McGEE

My life was on repeat. I was exhausted and depressed again and it was the postpartum. It had returned. This time I knew what it was and was more familiar with the symptoms. My doctors failed me again, they never offered me meds or even suggested I seek therapy. I was a young African American woman, they didn't care. I remember one day I felt so overwhelmed. I had the laundry bag in one hand, a diaper bag in another, all while juggling a car seat and trying to grab my eldest's hand. I felt like turning on the oven and not waking up. My only concern was leaving my babies and I kept thinking back to the time when my mom told me that "One day, those boys are going to grow up to take care of you, it won't always be like this." They were my reason why!

It was my last year at Elgin, a semester before graduation. I was working at the student minority office, with Mr. Melvin Scott. He asked me "What's next, what do you plan on doing after graduation?" I told him that I wanted to finish my education and he offered me an invite to a college tour which I graciously accepted. On the college tour, Mr. Scott exposed me to something I had never experienced before after becoming a mom. He gave me hope. He showed me that I can still be successful and go on to finish my education even with my two boys. I learned of family housing and applied for the fall. After getting accepted, my children and I were off to SIUC (Southern Illinois University of Carvondale) to start our new life.

Carvondale allowed me to walk by blind faith. I had never been so far away from my parents and was alone for the first time. Even though I quickly adjusted and got accumulated with my new schedule, It was still hard work. I had to juggle classes, be a mom, handle all of my kids activities and also work a full time job and an internship. My mornings started very early, considering I was dressing for three. Days were long, with me balancing my classwork and my internship and fortunately, I was able to get my kids into an extended daycare. Some days, I had to figure out how my sons could still be active in the sports they participated in such as t-ball, gymnastics and tai kwon doe.

Although my parents were farther away, they still remained very supportive. They paid my car note and still kept the boys, my paw-paw taking them to the country with him every summer. I don't know how I did it or where I got the strength from but I managed being a mom, and also having a social life. That next semester, my parents kept the boys so that I could live on campus and experience living in a dorm room. I would travel back to Chicago every weekend to visit my boys. Although I appreciated my parents for keeping them, I missed their presence too much. I was a mom! Needless to say, them being away and me living on campus only lasted that semester.

College was great. Even though I was a mom, it was the best years of my life. My children went to class with me and social gatherings. They basically grew up on campus and we grew up together. I applied for grad school at SIU, along with some other schools. I got accepted to Aurora University Social Work Masters Program. I moved back to my parents home for 2 months, until my apartment was ready. Life was good. I had learned how to be a parent to my children with little to no support from J. One day I got a call that he was arrested. I don't even know all the details because at the time we weren't in amicable space. My oldest son was 6 and he's now about to be 29, and his dad is still incarcerated. It's like a curse; my sons had to grow up without their dad just like I did. My biological dad got incarcerated again when I was 26 and there he remains.

My masters program was a one year program at Carol's Stream. I went to class, taking my boys with me and keeping them entertained while focusing on the lectures. One day, as I was leaving class, I ran into a military recruiter. He talked to me about the Air Force, and because I didn't have a plan after finishing grad school, it sounded really good to graduate and become an officer in the military. After graduation, I got a job and worked for Chicago public schools but going to the military always remained in the back of my head. After some time, I decided to go back to that same recruiters office, and I signed up for the Air Force. I left my boys for 3 months with my parents, and came back and worked as an Airmen.

My decision to go to the military was based off of me craving stability and the fact that they were willing to pay off my student

LAKEISHA McGEE

loans, not to mention all the great benefits for the boys and I. After serving 6 years in the military, I didn't re-enlist which I often regret not making a career out of it. The boys would spend the summer in Missouri with my dad and while I was at one of my duty stations, I received a call that my sons had been hit by a car and had to be airlifted to Memphis. After attempting to get in touch with the officer in command to no avail, I went AWOL.

The boys had been riding their bikes and a car turned the corner and hit them so hard that they flew in the air almost touching the electrical wires. My paw-paw watched all of this and told me he felt so helpless and was scared cause he thought my sons were dead. They had to be airlifted to Memphis Tennessee, Children's hospital. My oldest son's ribs were bruised very badly, almost broken. My youngest son had a broken collar bone, along with both knees, ribs and hips all broken. For the next 9 months he would be in a body cast, had to have rods put in both legs, underwent several blood transfusion surgeries and also having to attend physical therapy. The effects of the car accident caused my family to seek therapy. The trauma of the accident created PTSD for us all.

That summer, we took time to heal. Family therapy, family outings, and lots of doctors appointments. We started a family business, and I dabbled into real estate. We took every event that happened in our lives and made it a teachable moment, including the painful ones. As the summer progressed, so did the challenges of being a single parent. I was working a full time job, running the real estate business, and caring for both of my sons; one who could do nothing for himself. He was in a body cast and then eventually transitioned to a wheelchair once we began to attend physical therapy where he had to literally learn to walk again. He was such a strong kid.

Becoming a single teenage mother, was only one of the many adversities I would face throughout my life. I would later be in an abusive marriage, and then win a battle with breast cancer. Overcoming all of those things, took a lot of willpower, faith, and courage. Paw-paw always told me, I could do anything I wanted to do. He believed in me, and always encouraged me. As a result of that, I finished college with honors, have two master's degrees, completed my phd, have owned several small businesses including a non -profit. I have also had the honor of raising four beautiful children and most recently, I found out I was going to be a Mi'Ma.

Life has taught me some valuable lessons and being a single mother has taught me how to smash through brick walls. Some of the lessons I've learned are;
Before making a connection with a human being, get to know yourself first, then your partner.
Hard work pays off. Do what you have to do now, so you can do what you want to do later.
Trust the process, even when it's uncomfortable.
Trust yourself.
The most important lesson is to just keep going.
Build your team, meaning build your support system.
Set boundaries and goals and stick to them.
We often wonder why we're dealt certain cards in life, but nobody life is perfect. When given lemons, make lemonade.

DEDICATION

Agape love is described as a selfless, sacrificial and unconditional love. There is no greater form of love than that of agape. It is pure, genuine and everlasting. It's the kind of love that a mama bear has for her cubs!

Thank you Jason, Jordan, Journi and Jouris for choosing means doing this thing called life with me!

Thank you Mom for teaching me how to be the best mama bear there is.
Thank you PawPaw for choosing us to love. I survived it all because of your love. Without it, I am nothing!

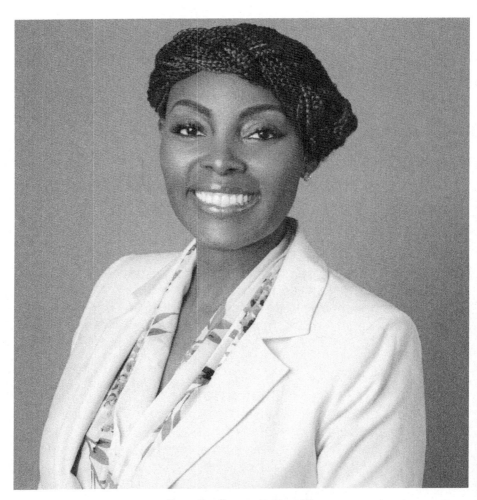

Lakeisha McGee

Lakeisha McGee

LaKeisha S. McGee has over 20 years of clinical experience in therapy, life coaching, and education. She's a specialist that teaches healing through the power of the Metanoia Method. Lakeisha's dedication to the enhancement and development of the complete person has motivated her to expand her knowledge base in the areas of intentional personal healing, community and most recently breast cancer advocacy.

On November 7, 2018, Lakeisha was diagnosed with Stage 2A Grade 7 Breast Cancer Her2+ Estrogen+, Progesterone+. That moment would change her life forever and create her new normal. This experience encouraged her to create HealHer2 Foundation. This foundation collaborates with others to create lasting partnerships that assist survivors affected by life-altering circumstances.

Prior to the creation of HealHer2 Foundation, Lakeisha worked for Chicago Public Schools for over 16 years serving in several different roles including Social Worker and Assistant Principal. Her ability to develop curriculum has afforded her the opportunity to create several programs for Chicago Public Schools, Safe Haven Summer Program and Mentoring Young Mothers of Greater DuPage Program (MYM).

Lakeisha has spoken for several organizations, Salvation Army, Georgia State University, Department of Children and Family Services and Susan G. Komen where she serves as an ambassador. Lakeisha McGee is also an international speaker she has spoken for the Ignite International Interview Series.

Lakeisha holds a BSW from Southern Illinois University in Carbondale, an MSW from Aurora University, an M.Ed from Lewis University and Ph.D from Concordia University. Some of her current research interests are human development through life coaching, community restoration by means of healing and accountability, human trafficking, and breast cancer awareness. Her most recent written work is an anthology, entitled 12 Shades of Breast Cancer. Lakeisha is a mother of four beautiful children and able to say she beat cancer...she's a Survivor!

WEB LINKS.
Website: https://lakeishamcgee.com/
Twitter: @specialistmcgee
LinkedIn: linkedin.com/in/lakeishamcgee

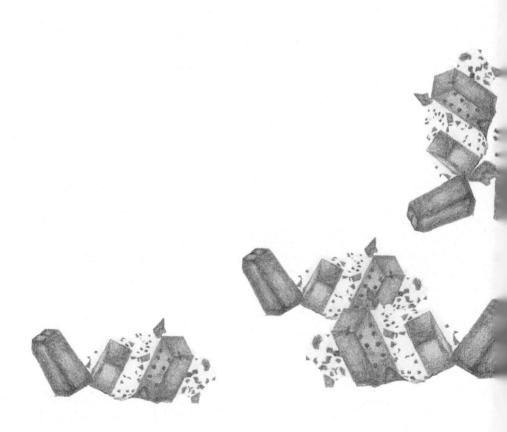

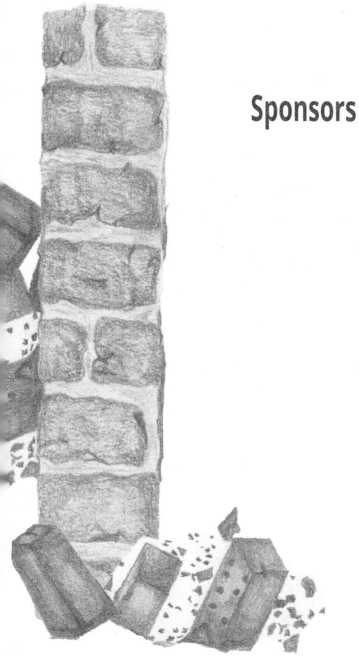

Sponsors

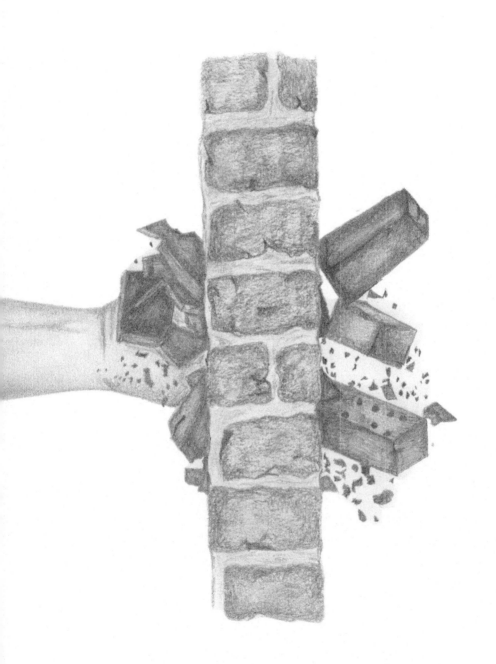

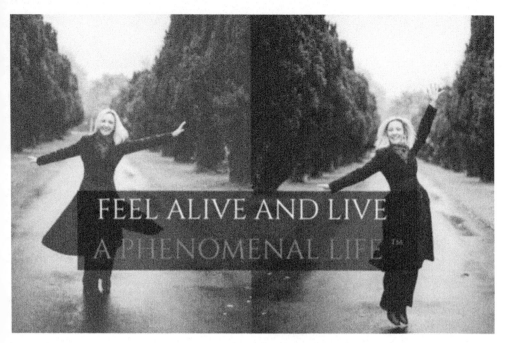

FEEL ALIVE AND LIVE
A PHENOMENAL LIFE™

Rebecca offers a huge range of opportunities to work with her to empower yourself with all areas of your life and business through her online digital programs, private bespoke coaching and much more.

Rebecca loves to share her highly positive energy with as many people around the world and if you stay with her long enough, she'll inspire and motivate you and empower your mindset so you know that you can achieve anything.

Available at all different price points you can tap into Rebecca's work at whatever level you are at too.
Connect with her on her website below.

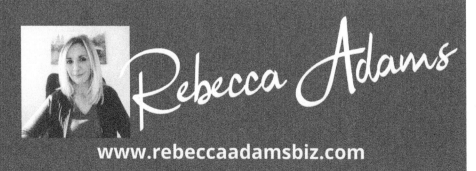

Rebecca Adams

www.rebeccaadamsbiz.com

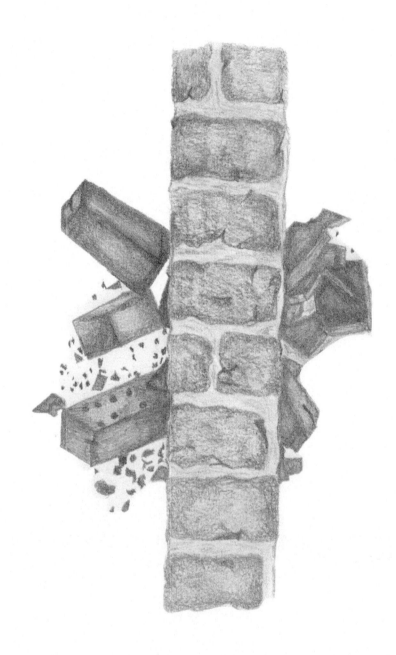

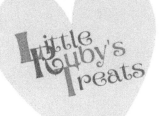

We are a small independent business offering Printing Services, Sweet gifts, mug hampers and hampers, all for a variety of occasions.
Our product range will continue to grow as our business grows.

All our products can be personalised or one of our generic designs
depending on your requirements.

We launched Little Ruby's Treats in 2021 with hopes and dreams that the business will grow steadily and become the company we envision it to be. We strive to offer a professional, friendly service and hope we will become your new favourite go to place for all your treats and gifts.

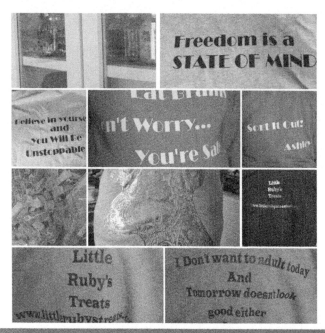

www.littlerubystreats.co.uk

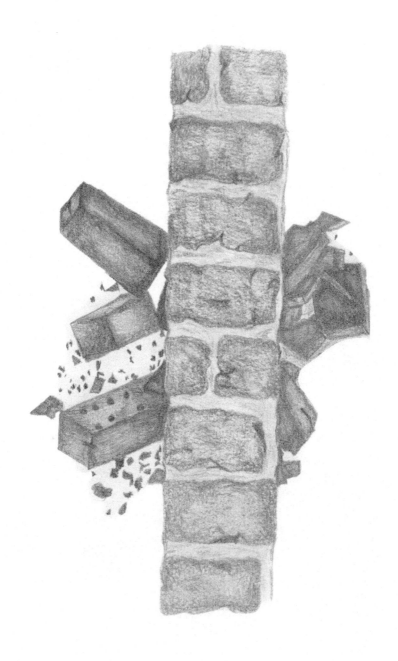

Write To Release
Journal & Pen

The "Write to Release" journal has been created as an outlet to release your feelings and emotions in a safe positive way when things become overwhelming; It is so important for our wellbeing and mental health to be able to feel free to release those feelings.

Using your voice is the best way to talk about what you may be going through but for those who find that challenging the next best thing is to write it down.

The written word can be very powerful and empowering especially when it is your written words, and can also be very healing; No one should ever feel afraid to release the things that no longer serve them.

Always be kind to yourself and know that you are enough.

Love and blessings
Jenny x

The Journal contains 215 pages, including affirmations, gratitude list, mindfulness colouring, and a creative space to draw, doodle, stick pictures in and use as a vision board.

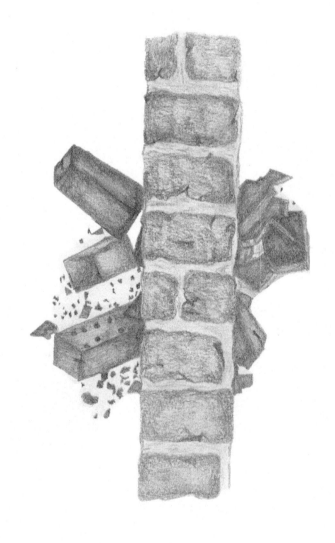

Thank You

Thank you kindly for choosing our book. The journey of collaborating with other Co-Authors across the U.S. and Internationally has been such a great experience both personally and professionally. Together we share a mutual understanding of True stories of abuse, tragedy and heartache leading to strength, hope and happiness.

I'd like to personally thank each co-author for putting their trust in me directing this endeavor and collectively making our voices heard!

Rebecca Adams

'In Loving Memory'

Carole Arnold.
July 1949 - April 2021.

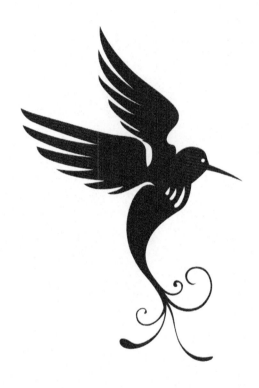

"She made broken look beautiful and strong look invincible.
She walked with the universe on her shoulders and made it
look like a pair of wings."

I know you are listening from above...

Love you our UK Mum
Irene xoxox

Printed in Great Britain
by Amazon

60949403R00119